The Social Value of Drug Addicts

MERRILL SINGER AND J. BRYAN PAGE

The
SOCIAL VALUE
of
DRUG ADDICTS
THE USES OF THE USELESS

WALNUT CREEK
CALIFORNIA

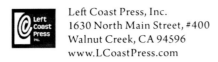
Left Coast Press, Inc.
1630 North Main Street, #400
Walnut Creek, CA 94596
www.LCoastPress.com

ISBN 978-1-61132-117-3 hardback
ISBN 978-1-61132-118-0 paperback
ISBN 978-1-61132-119-7 institutional eBook
ISBN 978-1-61132-751-9 consumer eBook

Library of Congress Cataloging-in-Publication Data

Singer, Merrill.
   The social value of drug addicts : uses of the useless / Merrill Singer, J Bryan Page.
     pages cm
   Summary: "Drug users are typically portrayed as worthless slackers, burdens on society, and just plain useless—culturally, morally, and economically. By contrast, this book argues that the social construction of some people as useless is in fact extremely useful to other people. Leading medical anthropologists Merrill Singer and J. Bryan Page analyze media representations, drug policy, and underlying social structures to show what industries and social sectors benefit from the criminalization, demonization, and even popular glamorization of addicts. Synthesizing a broad range of key literature and advancing innovative arguments about the social construction of drug users and their role in contemporary society, this book is an important contribution to public health, medical anthropology, popular culture, and related fields"—Provided by publisher.
   Includes bibliographical references and index.
   ISBN 978-1-61132-117-3 (hardback)
   ISBN 978-1-61132-118-0 (paperback)
   ISBN 978-1-61132-119-7 (institutional ebook)
   ISBN 978-1-61132-751-9 (consumer eBook)
   1. Drug addicts.   2. Social values.   3. Drug abuse—Social aspects.   I. Page, J. Bryan, 1947–   II. Title.
   HV5801.S48 2013
   305.9'084—dc23
                                                                                                 2013029130
Printed in the United States of America

Cover design by Martin Hoyem
Cover image: World Health Organization photo by C. Blackwell. Images from the History of Medicine, National Library of Medicine, PP044736 WHO box 3, Record 101437129.

CONTENTS

INTRODUCTION

> Casual drug users should be taken out and shot.
>> *Daryl Gates, former police chief, LAPD,*
>> *(quoted in Ostrow: 1990)*

> By World War I the American addict was identified as a social menace and equated with the IWWs [Industrial Workers of the World], Bosheviks, anarchists, and other fear subgroups
>> *David Musto, psychiatrist and drug historian, 1987*

> The fact that these really are the excess people in America, we—our economy doesn't need them.... We pretend that we're actually including them in the American ideal, but we're not. And they're not foolish. They get it.
>> *David Simon, producer of The Wire, 2008*

This book explores a prevailing and consequential contradiction of modernity. In diverse and interconnected arenas, from everyday popular discourse, to multiple sectors of the mass media and culture industries, to government pronouncements and reports, and to legislative exchange and court rulings, drug users routinely are portrayed as worthless slackers, evil doers, and lurking threats to the quality of life if not to the very survival of civil society—in short, as outcast Social Others with no positive value or useful contribution to society, the human rubbish of contemporary social life (Friedman 1998). As Taylor (2008:382) stresses

> [T]he news media and criminal justice policy seemingly mirror each other's beliefs. Indeed the reinforcement and belief in stereotypes and "outsiders" seems to be part of what appears to be a mutually beneficial partnership. "Drug stories (embellished with commonplace mythology) help sell papers." ... Especially drug stories which maintain and reinforce dominant and stereotypical images of drugs, drug users and drug-related crime.

Drug users are, it would seem, as David Simon brands them, excess people in America, a group of individuals that comprise a hollow surplus in our economy and a despised burden on society. But are drug users as socially worthless as they are portrayed?

The Social Value of Drug Addicts: The Uses of the Useless, by Merrill Singer and J. Bryan Page, 7–24. © 2014 Left Coast Press, Inc. All rights reserved.

Unpacking dominant ideologies about drug users in contemporary society, assessing the actual social roles of drug users, and questioning the social utility of depicting drug users as valueless (in both senses, as having no social worth and as lacking values) are the goals of this book. This volume seeks to address four interrelated questions, the first three of which are: (1) What are the reigning images of drug users in the modern world across assorted social domains and in the popular imaginary? (2) Are these portraits objective representations of drug users as they live their day-to-day lives, seemingly physically in but not culturally a part of society? and (3) How do we account for discrepancies between image and actual, between what anthropologists traditionally called the ideal (how we think social things should be) and the real (how social things actually are). Ultimately, answering these questions raises a fourth unifying query: What are the uses of the useless? Put differently, why (and to whom) is it useful to have some people defined as socially devoid of value? Although the answers to the first three of these questions are presented in this and the chapters that follow, the last question is addressed in the conclusion.

TEXTUAL CONSTRUCTION OF OUTSIDERS

Exemplary of the outcast motif are government-funded renderings of drug users and their adverse impact on the nation. In a speech given at the Heritage Foundation (Hutchinson 2002), the director of the Drug Enforcement Administration (DEA) stated

> Drug abusers become slaves to their habits. They are no longer able to contribute to the community. They do not have healthy relationships with their families. They are no longer able to use their full potential to create ideas or to energetically contribute to society, which is the genius of democracy. They are weakened by the mind-numbing effects of drugs. The entire soul of our society is weakened and our democracy is diminished by drug use.

Added Thomas Harrington (2011), while Assistant Administrator and Chief of Operations of the DEA, "[d]rug trafficking and abuse exact a significant toll on the American public. More than 38,000 Americans—or approximately 12 times the number of people killed by terrorists on September 11, 2001—died in 2007 as a direct result of the use of illicit drugs." Further, the DEA stresses, in addition to the many health and social problems experienced by drug users themselves, those who suffer at their hands include their families, the medical system, the environment. Innocent kids, caught in the crossfire. Drivers killed or injured by those under the influence. Babies found at meth labs, their toys covered with chemicals. Victims of terrorists, whose acts are financed with drug profits.... Direct costs include those for drug treatment, health care, costs of goods and services lost to crime, law enforcement, incarceration, and the judicial system fees. Indirect costs are those due to the loss of productivity from death, human suffering, drug abuse-related illnesses, victims of crime (Benavidez 2013:20)

In fact, if alcohol and tobacco were included as drugs in the calculation cited above, rather than just those drugs that have come to be banned in the United States, the actual figure in this emotionally charged statement would be 184 times greater than the number of those who died on September 11 (Mokdad et al. 2004) and the list of "other victims" would be even longer (e.g., cancer patients, those who suffer from diseases due to exposure to second-hand smoke, victims of fires sparked by cigarettes). As this carefully wrought distinction suggests, a critical aspect of constructing drug users as Others involves labeling; in this highly political activity some users of psychotropic drugs are included and denigrated as dangerous outsiders while others are excluded and protected from such representation (Becker 1963).

Othering processes are embedded in and propelled by language. As Haig Bosmajian notes in his book *The Language of Oppression* (1983:6), "While names, words and language can be and are used to inspire us, to motivate us to humane acts, to liberate us, they can also be used to dehumanize human beings and to 'justify' their suppression and even their extermination." Thus, with reference to the demonization of Jews, he notes that the Nazis' "persistent portrayal of the Jews as 'vermin,' 'bacilli,' 'parasites,' and 'disease' contributed to the 'Final Solution'" (Bosmajian 1983:8). The words and metaphors used to create distinction were referred to by Bosmajian as the "language of oppression." This is the language that characterizes much of the popular discourse on drug users.

Although written over 50 years ago, Howard Becker's (1953, 1955) early studies of marihuana use and his larger examination of marihuana users and musicians, entitled *Outsiders: Studies in the Sociology of Deviance* (Becker1963), remain highly relevant to efforts to understand linguistic processes of social labeling. According to Becker, deviance is not a quality of individuals, it is a product of social decisions. Deviance is not, in other words, an activity engaged in by terrible individuals but rather the outcome of someone with the power to do so publicly labeling someone's else's behavior as bad and acting on this accusation (including trying to convince those who are labeled that they are to blame for the punishment they receive). In the case of marihuana users, Becker described how during the 1930s the Federal Bureau of Narcotics flooded the mass media with alarming stories of marihuana-crazed Mexican immigrants, marihuana-induced rape and prostitution, and unsuspecting youth driven by marihuana use to a life of delinquency. Repeated media depictions of the social threat presented by marihuana users facilitated the passage of anti-marihuana laws (discussed in Chapter 6) while fixing in the popular imagination an image of drug consumers that had little to do with actual drug-related behavior and a lot to do with reinforcing social inequalities and controls.

A similar argument is made by Craig Reinarman and Harry Levine (1997) in their documentation of the series of "drug scares" that have spread in inundating social waves across the United States dating back to the temperance movement and its depictions of "demon alcohol." Such scares, they argue, characterized by "extraordinary antidrug frenzy," are driven by outrageous claims and "lurid stories about a new 'epidemic'; or 'plague' of drug use" (Reinarman and Levine 1997:1). Often these social upheavals occur independent of actual increases in drug use or evidence of mounting drug-related health and social problems.

Another, classic article, Alfred Lindesmith's (1940) "Dope Fiend Mythology," early on pointed out the existence of a body of stereotyped misinformation about drug addicts that was promoted by sensational articles and newspaper accounts. Found in these media depictions were routine accounts of the 'dope-crazed killer' and the 'dope-fiend rapist.' Notes Lindesmith (1940:199):

> The fact that the monstrous persons depicted exist mainly as figments of the imagination does not alter the fact that this mythology plays an important role in determining the way in which drug addicts are handled. Among serious students of the problem and among others who have some actual first hand contact with drug users, as for example prison officials, it has always been recognized that the American public is singularly misinformed on this subject. Nevertheless, the organization of the machinery of justice that deals with this problem is more directly based upon the superstitions of the man on the street than it is upon anything that has been done in the name of impartial and objective analysis.

In light of this analysis, Lindesmith (1940:208) came to believe that "treatment of addicts in the United States today is on no higher plane than the persecution of witches of other ages, and like the latter it is to be hoped that it will soon become merely another dark chapter of history."

A newspaper editorial written 70 years after Lindesmith's strident call for change suggests there has been little improvement in the way drug users are portrayed. Entitled "Drug Users Share the Blame in Officer's Death," it ran on January 5, 2009 in the *Dallas Morning News* (2009). In the view of the newspaper's editors, in light of the shooting death of police officer Cpl. Norman Smith during a drug raid in Dallas the prior day, everyone who uses illicit drugs, even occasional users, "have blood on [their] hands." When police officers are killed trying to control the flow of drugs, asserts the editorial, it is those who buy drugs that have put police in harm's way. Issues of compulsivity of addiction, the nature of policing practices, and the social enactment of policies that produce such raids are not discussed in the editorial, as the primary goal is to assign blame for the death of a policeman on all drug users everywhere and to make sure it is known that the newspaper "stands" with the family of the fallen officer.

In parallel fashion, in accounting for escalating drug-related violence in Mexico, Patrick Osio (2008) of New America Media, firmly asserts that it is time to "take the gloves off and lay the responsibility for the bloodbath taking place on a daily basis in Mexico where it belongs—U.S. drug users." Those liable for the fact that "Mexican-style mafiosos are killing each other along with Mexican police officers, judges, prosecutors, journalists and innocent bystanders—be they adults or children" (Osio 2008) are those in the United States who buy small quantities of Mexican drugs on local street corners in L.A. or Chicago. Again, the fact that the National Institute on Drug Abuse defines drug addiction in medical terms and not as personal moral failing, or that illicit drug corporations and mainstream legal corporations are often extensively intertwined (e.g., bank laundering of drug money), or that it is unlikely that illicit drugs would flow as readily to American cities without police corruption are not addressed by Osio.

IMAGING AND THE IMAGINARY

Cultural meanings and messages are not conveyed by words alone. Images are equally if not more influential in fixing dominant understandings. As Ross (2011a:5) indicates, "the power and utility of images to inscribe concepts into the minds of readers and viewers" rests in their direct communication without the ambiguities of words. Consider the cultural blackening of poverty in the United States. Even without the urgency of a sudden catastrophe like Hurricane Katrina or the sober shadow of an immediate calamity in the hotly contested politics of everyday life, there is a tendency in the United States to blur negative images resulting in the poor being presented pictorially as African American or another socially devalued ethnic group, and ethnic minorities, in turn, being visually portrayed as drug-using threats to the white middle class. The process through which this image construction takes place is seen, for example, in Steven Gregory's 1996 ethnographic study of Lefrak City, a predominantly African American apartment complex in Queens County, New York. Gregory (1996:35) found that, despite available data that contradicts such portrayals, in nearby primarily white neighborhoods Lefrak City is imagined and visualized as "a site of danger, decay, and dirt-images linked symbolically with pollution and disorder...." These constructions, in turn, Gregory (1996:24) observes, are based on fixed images of the apartment complex as a center of "black crime, poverty, and drugs—a racialized threat to the area's quality-of-life and a [necessary] focus of law enforcement and neighborhood 'stabilization' strategies."

The theory of hegemony developed by Antonio Gramsci (1971) is particularly relevant to assessing the role of images in the ingraining of cultural stereotypes in the media and other dominant social institutions. Gramsci engaged the question of why, given their exploitation, were the working classes of Europe prior to World War II not more revolutionary in their orientation and even open to the anti-working class ideas of fascism? The reason, Gramsci argued, was because dominance is not maintained through outright physical force but through mechanisms that persuade subordinate classes to accept the moral, political and cultural values of the dominant group. These class-based values form part of a cultural universe in which all classes are socialized and experience the world. As Gramsci stressed, television, the movies, and other everyday sources of popular images function as critical engines in the ongoing reproduction of hegemony. Such images, linking minorities or the poor with violence, sexuality, drug use, or other threatening behaviors, are part and parcel of the process through which people assimilate attitudes about drug users. Based on his experience working at the BBC, Tony Freeth (1985:26-27), producer and director of the Campaign Against Racism in the Media, notes

> It all takes place in an atmosphere of smiling, middle-class gentility, an air of righteous indignation if confronted with charges of racism. No

one in TV shouts racist abuse at black people.... No one in TV physically assaults black people, they simply feed us on a diet of "Blacks are the problem."

As a result of the ingrained and representational nature of hegemonic messages there has been a failure to recognize that the media serves purposes beyond entertainment or narrow educational goals in terms of particular broad and naturalized understandings of the world. Central to this understanding is the routine acceptance of white privilege. According to Lipsitz (1995:369), "As the unmarked category against which difference is constructed, whiteness never has to speak its name, never has to acknowledge its role as an organizing principle in social and cultural relations." Moreover, of equal importance in the hegemonic messages of the media are affirmations of the intellectual and moral superiority of the elite sectors of society and the utter intellectual, moral, economic, and social depravity of drug users.

One of the mechanisms through which popular thinking about drug users is periodically reinforced is through the media generation of "moral panics" (Cohen 1995). These commonly entail the media discovery of a new drug or drug form, exaggerated and distorted portrayals of the drugs harmful effects, and growing emphasis on the threat to society presented by the new drug's users. In this way, drugs are invested with the symbolic power to instigate popular moral indignation while overtly or covertly indicating the need for greater social control to protect society from the emergent danger. As Mcdermott (1992) observes,

[A] media-driven moral panic emerges from a systematic world view based upon an imaginary consensus that governs all reporting. This portrays the world as bifurcated into certain binary oppositions, e.g., Normal/Deviant, Sick/Wicked, Corrupt/Innocent.

Young (1973) adds that the portrayal of drug users by the media is so consistently misinformed, sensationalized, and inaccurate that it would seem that journalists lack access to the subjects of their accounts, which, as anthropologists who have long studied street drug users, we know is certainly not the case. Rather, as Mcdermott (1992) concludes, "the systematic nature of this type of coverage implies that the origins of this portrayal has its place in the social structure," an argument that is central to this volume.

The sources of the depictions of drug users that feed the popular imagination are varied. Carl Hart, a neuroscientist at Columbia University, has investigated the behavioral and neuropharmacological effects of psychotropic drugs in the laboratory by making available crack cocaine and methamphetamine to active users and testing for factors that mediate drug self-administration behavior. To Hart's surprise, documented in his personal account, *High Price: A Neuroscientist's Journey of Self-Discovery That Challenges Everything You Know About Drugs and Society* (Hart 2013), his research findings did not match the expectations he had about drug users based on his exposure to them through the diverse sectors of the media. This understanding of crack and meth users, Hart (2013:2–3) notes, included the belief that:

> No matter what, they'd do anything to get to take as much drugs as often as possible. I thought of them in the disparaging ways I'd seen them depicted in films like New Jack City and Jungle Fever and in songs like Public Enemy's "Night of the Living Baseheads." ... Back then I believed that drug users could never make rational choices, especially about their drug use, because their brains had been altered or damaged by drugs.

Yet Hart found his research participants did make rational decisions and, further, did not live up to any of the established and widely broadcast popular understandings about hardcore drug users.

> Over and over, these drug users continued to defy conventional expectations. Not one of them crawled on the floor, picking up random white particles and trying to smoke them. Not one was ranting or raving. No one was begging for more, either—and absolutely none of the cocaine users I studied ever became violent. I was getting similar results with methamphetamine users. They, too, defied stereotypes (Hart 2013:3).

Experiences like these led Hart to consider alternative explanations of the behaviors often assigned to drug abusers, an examination that brought him to the conclusion that the effects of structural violence, including poverty, discrimination, and social marginalization, have been misrepresented as the effects of drug use.

As we show in this volume, beyond (or usually intertwined) with descriptive and categorizing words are socially useful pictorial representations of drug users, both those that are channeled to the public (as well as policy makers and the workforces of social-control institutions) via the media, including still photographs (e.g., in the print and electronic news media) and moving pictures (e.g., TV news, television and movie dramas, video, and documentaries), and those that become established in people's minds and memories, are consequential cultural products. In her analysis of wedding photographs in Taiwan, for example, Adrian (2003:19) refers to pictures as "circulating visual texts" that are "rich with cultural meanings and textured by social relationships." This is no less true with regard to pictures and visual portrayals of drug users. Routinely, images of drug users carry a dual message of menace and mystery. They are depicted as being at once dangerous to others and to themselves. Not only do family and friends as well as strangers suffer at their hands, their self-inflicted emotional and physical wounds are portrayed as especially deep and damaging. Such imagery affirms "the power of pictures" to influence lives. (Elliot 2011).

Generally, media depictions of drug users, comprising "a shorthand to telegraph blunt, … stereotypical messages," constitute "images that injure" (Ross 2011a:5). Despite this harm, experienced daily by drug users in their interactions with other sectors of society, the pictorial manufacture of drug user stereotypes continues because it is useful. As Ross (2011b:1) stresses, despite dramatic changes in the composition of media venues in recent years, the media remains "a vital cog in the capitalist machine in the United States and around the world," and as such it generally tends "to reproduce, redistribute, and magnify the powerful messages and images from the very few who control the purse strings of the major media conglomerates."

As Hickman (2009) has argued, there has been a relentless process of envisioning drug users and addiction over the last 120 years. As a result of such images in the media and elsewhere, "Everyone knows what a junkie is supposed to look like: hollow cheeks, panda eyes, haunted expression, wasted, decadent, desperate" (Hickman 2009:119). Such images showed up boldly, for example, in advertisements and glossy fashion magazines during the 1990s in a style that came to be known as Heroin-Chic (Ehrman 1995, Halnon 2009). But this was but one moment in a much longer cultural concern with "our overwhelming desire to look" at drug users in the media, in art, in film, in social science texts, and elsewhere (Hickman 2009:136). As we gaze "with fascination, revulsion or romantic longing at pictures of narcotics addicts trapped in their own downward spiral, we ultimately confront our own obsessions and the need to feed them with an endless supply of satisfactory visual stimuli (Hickman 2009:136). This too is one of the multiple uses of the useless.

OTHERING AND STIGMATIZATION

The textual and visual social construction of drug users, involving "technologies of exclusion" (Anselmi and Gouliamos 1998) in various representation forms, constructs them not only as different but as useless, and all that that understanding of them implies in terms of the ways they are treated in society, as well as their own internalized self-images, rests on processes of distinction and ranking. Distinction is a cultural practice that divides things in the world on the basis of socially meaningful criteria and differentially values some over others based on alleged distinctive capacities. When applied to people, processes of distinction have been referred to as Othering (Riggins 1997), which entails a two-step progression involving, first, the binary act of inclusion (seeing one's own perceived social group as "us") and exclusion (seeing other identified groups as "them"), and second, the ethnocentric affirmation of one's own group as normal through the denigration of other groups as abnormal. As Labute (2004:71–72) stresses:

> People are not comfortable with difference.... The thing [people seen as different] represent that's so scary is what we could be, how vulnerable we all are.. ..We're all just one step away from what being what frightens us. What we despise. So ... we despise it when we see it in anybody else.

Othering, in short, entails the "assertion of difference as deficit" (Schwalbe et al. 2002:423).

As a core organizing practice in the creation and maintenance of social inequality, a dominant feature of modern society, Othering is comprised of a suite of behavioral practices by in-groups, including stereotypic thinking, stigmatizing marking and bounding, social distancing, dehumanization, justification of oppressive dominant practices, and (possibly) commodification of outgroups (Lister 2004). Each of these will be discussed in turn.

Stereotypic thinking involves the assumption that all members of a group are more or less the same; they all share a set of inherent traits that are alternatively valued (i.e., our traits) or devalued (i.e., their traits). As Lee (1989:10) emphasizes, stereotypic thinking tends to be "unchanging, rigid, overly categorical, undifferentiated, ... overly simplistic, and inaccurate because variation among individual instances is not taken into account," among other reasons. In the case of drug users in modern society, individual personality and behavioral differences are erased and drug use (or addiction) and its presumed uniform effects are treated as the dominant characteristics of all members of this identified and devalued group (Schur 1971).

Marking and bounding are processes of identifying distinctive badges of group membership (e.g., styles of dress, ways of talking, types of behavior, occupation of particular social spaces) for self and Others and the erection of largely impassable social barriers between groups (Fine 1994, Weis 1995). Marking and bounding commonly are expressions of stigmatization, which generally is understood in terms of Goffman's (1963:5) seminal discussion of this phenomenon as involving the social construction of "an undesired differentness" that engulfs the whole person and results in their discrediting and disempowerment relative to non-stigmatized individuals. Notable social markers of contemporary drug users include various psychiatric labels, such as impulsivity or addictive personality (e.g., Verdejo-Garcia, Lawrence and Clark 2008), particular forms of public appearance (e.g., inexpensive or worn clothing, a disheveled malnourished look, lack of self-care), specific identifying behaviors (e.g., being nervous, involvement in criminal activity), and being a member of an ethnic minority. As Bass and Kane-Williams (1993:79) reported with regard to the later point, "The picture most Americans have of a typical drug dealer or users is that of a young black male and the impression is that drug use is rampant and universal in the black community." Underlying these assumed traits, the stigmatization of drug users begins with their construction as amoral or immoral beings capable of the most heinous crimes imaginable. Such imagery remains despite studies clearly showing the regularity and normalization of drug use in particular populations, such as young adults (Blackman 2010; Parker, Aldridge, and Measham 1998, Parker, Williams and Aldridge 2002). One expression of the continued adverse effects of marking and bounding processes with drug users is seen in the limited availability of drug treatment. While lip service may be paid in public discourse to the need for more and better drug treatment, the directing of public funds to treatment (compared to the amount spent on interdiction, arrest, and incarceration of drug users), and the actual availability of and access to treatment, after care and social reintegration programs belies the existence of a strong social commitment to recovery from drug use (Singer 2004). Socially, in fact, there is a widespread (if inaccurate) assumption that drug use treatment does not work and hence it is a waste of public resources on an undeserving and recalcitrant population. Notes outspoken British judge Peter Moss

(Whitehead 2009), for example, "I can't think of any drug rehabilitation programmes that have been a success." As a result, pathways from drug use are narrow and drug users are seen as a dangerous group that must be kept away from society through the construction of a vast system for long-term incarceration. This attitude is found, as well, more broadly in the healing and criminal-justice professions. Baker and Isaac (1973:245), for example, found that the nurses, law students, and police they studied, "described drug abusers as immoral people committing an immoral act by taking drugs and as displaying criminal tendencies."

Social distancing, which follows from marking and boundary-making, entails the creation of guarded social space separating approved and disapproved groups. Note Nisim and Benjamin (2010:222), "The oppressive power of Othering is derived from the impassable barrier it forms between "us" and "them" and the social distancing it creates." The creation of social distance from drug users not uncommonly is propelled by fear, repugnance and repulsion. In a Tennessee study of attitudes toward drug addicts that including police trainees and college students who did not use drugs, for example, Doctor and Sieveking (1973:697) found that

> for the most part, policemen and nonusers saw the addict as having problems that were dissimilar to their own, repulsive and behaviorally unpredictable, and as requiring long-term assistance. Policemen felt significantly more strongly [than students] … that addicts … were not the type of people they would choose as close friends.

Further, as Kallen (1989) argues, social distancing of drug users is driven by a fear of contagion, a caricature that legitimizes discrimination, marginalization, pariahization, and dehumanization.

Dehumanization of drug users takes many forms, one critical one being the way they are treated by police. Describing the handling of inebriated Native Americans by off-reservation police, for example, Stratton (1973:615–616) observes:

> The treatment given drunks ranged from indifference to brutality. Among the policemen observed, callousness and impatience prevailed; rarely did they display any type of kind treatment. Several patrolmen occasionally employed verbal or physical abuse. Often they were curt; one patrolman tauntingly encouraged a woman getting out of the paddy wagon to fall on her face.

THE POLITICS OF DEMONIZATION

In the political consciousness and social ideologies that are forged through the intersection of media messages and images, official announcements, and community discursive activities, demonized understandings of drug users emerge that serve as a rationale not only for state punishment but for segregation, discrimination, and ethnic inequality as well (Mosher and Atkins 2007). In recent years, a significant influence on the development of this pattern was the announcement by President Ronald Reagan, in a major policy speech in 1986, calling for "a national crusade against drugs ... to rid America of this scourge" (quoted in Courtwright et al. 1989:344). There followed in subsequent years an ever-accelerating war on (primarily ethnic minority) drug users that has resulted in the annual arrest of over a million suspected drug offenders, most for simple drug possession or small-scale drug sale, and the rapid and dramatic escalation of the US prison population. As Dinglestad et al. (1996:1834) comment, "in the United States perhaps half of all current prisoners were convicted of drug offences or drug-related crimes.... Drug laws provide a convenient way to target certain groups: affluent drug users are seldom bothered by police, who concentrate more on poor, unemployed and minority groups." This approach sends a dual social message that is reinforced through multiple institutions in society, namely that drug users are dangerous and must put behind bars where they can do no harm and the poor and ethnic minorities use drugs and must be monitored and controlled.

The result is a frequently echoed social statement about drug users as human rubbish. Indeed, this is the very term for drug users and other devalued patients employed by the health care providers described by Roger Jeffery (1979) in his analysis of discrimination in hospital emergency rooms. Notes Jeffery (1979) "two broad categories were used to evaluate patients: good or interesting, and bad or rubbish." Various other demeaning labels are applied by health care workers to alcoholics and illicit drug users encountered as hospital patients. In the early 1980s, for example, Page heard emergency room staff at Jackson Hospital in Miami using the term "SHPOS" ("Sub-Human Piece of Shit") to refer to recidivistic alcoholics and heroin addicts who would present more than once during a three-month rotation. Other comparable labels include: "AALFD" ("Another Asshole Looking For Drugs"), "FD" ("Fucking drunk"), PG (Pharmaceutically Gifted), "SBOD" ("Stupid bitch/bastard on drugs"), "SHS" ("Sullen, Hostile, Stupid," which often is used specifically refer to an inner city drug/alcohol addict), and "PPA" (Practicing Professional Alcoholic).

These examples affirm the value of Murray Edelman's (1988:103) work on symbolic politics, including his understanding of the role of language as "the key creator of the social worlds people experience, not a tool for describing objective reality." Language in use, from this perspective, is a critical element in the social definition and construction of social problems. In this process, specific words (used both as "labels" of the problem that give it a distinct focus, and as descriptive and emotional "characterizers" of the nature and level of the social threat it poses) are mobilized in support of desired solutions. As Edelman argues, the latter often have already been selected by empowered social elites, based on their own ideologies and self-interested policy preferences, and language is identified to construct the social problem in a way that implies it is resolvable or at least governable by the selected control strategies. The adoption of elite solutions is facilitated by moral entrepreneurs skilled in the generation of public anxiety, if not outright moral panic, often through the use of mass media, and the manipulation of images of good and evil in the expressed defense of vital moral boundaries (Buchanan et al. 2003). Through the efforts of moral entrepreneurs, elite ideology is translated into symbolic crusades. As Gusfield (1963) indicates, symbolic crusades—moral campaigns to correct wayward behaviors waged by particular status groups within society against other social groups—ultimately reflect political controversies, assertions of authority, and exercises in the assertion of political power. Gusfield (1963:5) thus describes the initial development of the American temperance movement as "one way in which a ... social elite [the New England Protestant aristocracy] tried to retain ... its social power and leadership" relative to an emergent industrial working class. As temperance concerns spread to other parts of the country, other local social hierarchies came into play.

Moreover, as Yongming (1999) demonstrates in his analysis of 20th century anti-drug campaigns in China, symbolic crusades involve issues of governance and state building. Such campaigns, he argues, involve two components, hegemonic discourses and social and political practices. While serving the interests of economic and political elites, modern anti-drug crusades are primarily waged publicly by governments. Anti-drug crusades offer states a vehicle for asserting a particular worldview and social order (discourse) and a means of further consolidating power within society (practices).

Nowhere are these insights better illustrated than in the U.S. politics of crime and drug involvement during the past 20 years. One expression of the reigning narratives portraying drug users as ultimate moral threats to American society was the passage of draconian laws designed to punish severely those arrested for drug-related offenses. A prime example is the Supreme Court decision on June 27, 1997, upholding a Michigan state law that imposed a mandatory sentence of life in prison without possibility of parole for those convicted of possessing more than 1.5 pounds of cocaine. Through this decision the Supreme Court, as a branch of government, embraced the idea that having this amount of cocaine is the equivalent of the heinous crime of first-degree murder (the conscious and deliberate taking of a human life). Demonization of drug users in this instance served not only to enhance state power over the lives of those directly involved with illicit drugs, but, as a result of the social enforcement practices needed to identify, capture, and convict drug-related violators, the communities in which they live as well.

A further illustration of the dominant "blame drug users" mindset, one that gained national attention, was the explanation given by elected officials for the looting that occurred in New Orleans during the difficult days following Hurricane Katrina in 2005. With the city devastated, and many residents still stranded by polluted flood waters, the media began carrying sensational stories of widespread looting at local retail businesses. Shocking to many television viewers around the country was footage showing people using inflatable mattresses and other floatation devices to haul away stolen appliances, electronic gear, and other non-survival goods. According to New Orleans Mayor Ray Nagin, during an interview on Air America Radio, drug users were to blame for the looting and other violence in the struggling city (CNN.com 2005). In like manner, when interviewed on *The Early Show*, Louisiana Governor Kathleen Blanco at first insisted she was not going to play "the blame game," nonetheless she went on to assert that drug addicts were the main perpetrators of looting in the battered city. As the Drug Policy Alliance Network (2005) observed,

> This problem is, of course, not unique to New Orleans. All over the country substance abusers are routinely blamed for crime and other social ills—there is little discussion of the notion that prohibitionist drug policies themselves contribute to just these sorts of problems. It is far more politically popular to point to "drug addicts" as the bogeymen.

USES OF THE USELESS

Despite the routine and redundant depiction of drug users as wasted and worthless, closer examination reveals that they regularly are put to good social use in multiple ways, including, as discussed more thoroughly in the Conclusion, through the entertainment media as rich sources of dramatic distraction, as negative role models who help define the boundaries of approved behavior, as sources of very cheap labor (in and out of prison), as evidence of the unassailability of dominant understandings and values, and as conveniently scapegoated objects of blame for an array of social ills. In other words, this book, a product of many years of ethnographic research among drug users by its authors, is about the uses of the useless, the value of the devalued, and the meaning of those whose lives are represented as meaningless, wasted, and derelict.

The purpose of the book, in short, is demonstrate the accuracy of Edelman's (1988:103) observation that the language and related actions of official government sources, the mass media, the cultural industries, policy makers and enforcers, and even public health is "the key creator of the social worlds people experience, not a tool for describing objective reality." We seek to achieve this aim by dragging into clearer view the constructed nature of drug use and drug users as these are understood and responded to, especially in the United States, but elsewhere as well, and, through this analytic process, to cast a clarifying light on taken-for-granted assumptions, disguised but punishing inequalities and injustices, the aggrandizement of governmental power and corresponding restriction of rights and liberties accorded by the Constitution to the citizenry, and significant institutionalized mechanisms of everyday social control. Pursuing this objective entails an exploration of a phenomenon sociologist Lynn Zimmer (1992) termed "drugspeak." This term labels the existence of an anti-drug semantic that problematically but usefully constructs the nature of drug taking and the character of drug users. This construction, a component of a wider cultural war that is waged through multiple overlapping institutions, insures the dominance of a public attitude about drug users and their behavior that weds fear and loathing. As Gordon (1994) indicates, drugspeak

> establishes the legitimacy of law enforcement as the primary solution to the U.S. drug problem and endorses an unprecedented vigor and reach in applying criminal and civil penalties to those who defy prohibition.. ... Drugspeak suppresses all but the most academic discussion of policy alternatives, deflects attention from items on the shadow agenda of anti-drug activists, and prevents consideration of the structural sources of the most destructive forms of drug use.

HOLISM

A key insight of anthropology is that cultural systems are complex woven tapestries of interconnectedness and repetition. Central to the distinctive character of any "culture" are key themes that find expression across the various domains of social life, from politics to religion, from kinship to educational and enculturation processes, and from recreational activities to forms of social conflict. As Wolf (1982:388) explains, "The development of an overall hegemonic pattern or "design for living" [i.e., a "culture"] is not so much the victory of a collective cognitive logic or aesthetic impulse as the development of redundancy—the continuous repetition, in diverse instrumental domains, of the same basic propositions regarding the nature of constructed reality." Individualism, a core cultural code in American society, is reinforced through its repetitive expression in diverse domains, including the parceling out of food onto individual plates (as contrasted with shared group bowls or platters), the tendency to allow (except in the case of small children) only individual patients into the privacy of a physician's exam room, the expectation that individuals will put their personal career, employment, and other demands over the needs of parents and siblings (as contrasted with the familial concept of embedded identity as found in other "cultures"), and the constant pattern of individual assessment and ranking in work and other settings and the related heralding of personal achievement and accusation of individual failure.

Key cultural themes about drug users, and their social implications and uses, are explored in the following chapters across multiple cultural domains. Not surprisingly, in a complex cultural system like that found in Western societies, there are some arenas of contradiction and even conflict in the ways drug users are portrayed across domains. Still, the overwhelming slant is negative, harsh, and adversely consequential for drug users, while being beneficial for others who profit from drug-user demonization.

CONTENT

To achieve the critical aims outlined above, the book is organized into the following chapters. Chapter 1 examines the critical role race, class, and gender attitudes and hierarchies play in the social (mal)construction of drug users. The chapter examines the landscape of persons whose drug use defines them as deviant, while dismantling the highly complex and troubling (if socially useful) set of images that surround drug use. Chapters 2 and 3 provide historic depth to our examination, reviewing the origins and development of "drug use Otherness" by addressing the question: How did drug users come to be defined as deviant? Chapter 3, in particular, focuses on Prohibition and its enduring impacts. Subsequent chapters explore the images of drug use constructed in various sectors of society. Drug use and drug users in the world of literature is the focus of Chapter 4. Of concern is drug use by writers and literary writing about (or depicting) drug use, including autobiographical (or near-autobiographical) work. A similar approach is followed in Chapter 5, which looks at drug use and the movies. Chapter 6 addresses the legal construction of drug users, through drug laws, other policies, the courts, police practices, incarcerating institutions as well as the War on Drugs. Chapter 7 holds up a mirror to our own multidisciplinary field of social-science studies, the ways it has constructed drug users, and the benefits derived by researchers from having drug users as objects of study. In the Conclusion, we pull the threads of our argument together by addressing the myriad uses of the useless (for others with vested and self-serving interests) and the need for a radically different course in how we think about and behave toward people who consume drugs.

As drug researchers, we know about the ways drug users have been useful to us (as participants in our studies and as subjects in tests of prevention and intervention programs designed to address health risks drug users face). In examining the social, political, and communication mechanisms through which drug users come to endure suffering and mistreatment, we seek to be useful to them as an oppressed group. Our concern is with reducing the harm done to drug users by Othering and, ultimately, how this mistreatment adversely rebounds on society. In other words, we urge far-reaching change in a social arrangement in which we all—drug users and non-drug users alike—pay a cost so that some might benefit from the creation of a pariah group.

CHAPTER ONE

Drugs, Race, and Gender in the Social Construction of Drug Consumers

Recognizing the Origins of Othering

When human behavior involves the illicit ingestion of mind-altering drugs, the discourse about that behavior tends to accrue layers of social judgment, prejudice, stereotyping, and fear. This Othering process is hardly unexpected, given the personal experience that many people can claim as a result of having direct contact with drug-impaired people, but how much of it is "real" (i.e., in the sense of being empirically verifiable) and how much is constructed (i.e., based on culturally learned and socially motivated attitudes and beliefs)? Race, socioeconomic status, and gender constitute principal components of how people in the contemporary world perceive any complex of behaviors, and drug use is no exception. Basic prejudice against drug use and drug users tends to push perceptions in the direction of pejorative terms and discriminatory behavior.

These perceptions often rationalize and exacerbate racial and socioeconomic blame or gender prejudice. For example, the "typical" heroin user in some cities may be conceptualized as African American and may have traits attributed to him/her that correspond to racial stereotypes, such as unwillingness to work, irresponsibility, being given to larceny, and being dedicated to hedonistic pursuits. Although the literature lacks any definitive empirical data on the precise characteristics of the population of heroin users for the United States, the data contain sufficient basis to say that none of these stereotypes is true nationwide. White males dominate the population of heroin users, and some portion of this population, both African American and white, have regular jobs and families. The same applies to drug users of other ethnic identities as well. Along the lines of gender, in part females stand accused of heavy use of anti-anxiety medication (e.g., "mother's little helpers" as enshrined in the lyrics of a classic Rolling Stones song), stereotypically characterized as over-stressed housewives, desperate to keep all the plates of life spinning at once, worrying about their children and their future, and trying to please demanding and unappreciative husbands. The research data actually show, however, that relatively few women take minor tranquilizers regularly, and that their potential for addiction, although present, is not great. Nevertheless, stereotypes like this exist—in fact much harsher ones abound—and are perpetuated in the public imaginary.

What are the origins of these pejorative conceptualizations? Are they totally false, or do they contain a grain of truth? How do we go about discerning the difference between unwarranted assumptions about drug users and their "true nature?" Why do these harshly judgmental configurations populate media messages, inform (or misinform) public policy, and adversely impact the lives of many people? This chapter addresses these questions, while dismantling the highly complex and troubling (if socially useful) set of images that surround drug using behavior and characterize drug users as devalued people. Specifically, the chapter examines the social and media construction of the poor as an unworthy group of people in society, including exploration of the politically useful concepts of the "welfare queen" and "welfare cheaters" as tropes for people of color in efforts to gut welfare programs. Embedded in the perspectives that drive such efforts, the chapter argues, is the belief that many if not most welfare recipients use their benefits to buy drugs and get high. This linkage of poverty and drug abuse in contemporary thinking about people of color, has helped to promote the incarceral and anti-community policies of the War on Drugs, the multi-generation reproduction of an unequal opportunity structure, and the single-minded and simple-minded demonizing of illicit drug use (Reignarman and Levine 1997).

THE MAKING OF THE UNDESERVING POOR

During the 2012 presidential race, Republican candidate Mitt Romney gave a now infamous talk at a May 17 fundraiser in Boca Raton, Florida. Now known as the 47% speech (MoJo News Team 2012), Romney asserted the following:

> There are 47 percent of the people who will vote for the president no matter what. All right, there are 47 percent who are with him, who are dependent upon government, who believe that they are victims, who believe that government has a responsibility to care for them, who believe that they are entitled to health care, to food, to housing, to you name it. That that's an entitlement. And the government should give it to them. And they will vote for this president no matter what.... These are people who pay no income tax.

Reflected in this speech is a view of the poor, including poor working people, held by economic elites within society, a view that is disseminated to the society as whole through various communication media. This is the view that there are many undeserving poor, people who are a weight on society rather than contributors to it; moreover, they are said to rob society to the degree that they received any government-supported health or social program benefits. This view, as Navarro (1986:2) points out, is historically rooted in an "active ideological offensive [designed to] create a new consensus around a new set of values, beliefs and practices" regarding the poor. This perspective sees the poor as a form of dependent, defective, and delinquent social parasite.

Exemplary of this attitude is the pejorative term "welfare queen" which was introduced into the English language in 1976, primarily by Ronald Reagan. In his political speeches, Reagan built an image of poor people who feel entitled to the benefit of other people's hard work. He illustrated this claim using a newspaper report about a Chicago woman named Linda Taylor who was convicted of using various aliases and of cheating the government using false welfare applications. A parallel case even older than Taylor's is the so-called "lady in mink," as she was known after New York newspapers in 1947 printed several articles about a woman wearing a mink stole who showed up at a welfare office to pick up a check. Eventually, in this case, the *New Yorker*'s press critic A. J. Liebling (1947) revealed that despite having collected a large divorce settlement a number of years earlier, the woman and her 5-year old daughter were now dependent on $5.40 a day from the New York City welfare department. Moreover, the seemingly stylish mink was, in fact, old and deteriorating and of little real monetary value. This type of mischaracterization, as we will show, is the norm in this entire genre of attack narrative.

Being an accomplished storyteller (his nickname was the "Great Communicator"), and given to using stereotypes about the poor, on the campaign trail Reagan embellished the details of Linda Taylor's case, without actually using her name, to create a fictive individual whom he presented as both real and as representative of the undeserving, socially useless poor. Said Reagan (*New York Times* 1976) of a woman in Chicago:

> She has eighty names, thirty addresses, twelve Social Security cards and is collecting veteran's benefits on four non-existing deceased husbands. And she is collecting Social Security on her cards. She's got Medicaid, getting food stamps, and she is collecting welfare under each of her names. Her tax-free cash income is over $150,000.

All of this imagery was built on a relative minor case of welfare fraud involving about $8,000. In their book, "The Mommy Myth," Susan Douglas, a professor of communication studies at the University of Michigan, and Meredith Michaels, of the Department of Philosophy at Smith College (2004:185), pointed out the nature of Reagan's innovative stereotyping:

> He specialized in the exaggerated, outrageous tale that was almost always unsubstantiated, usually false, yet so sensational that it merited repeated recounting.... And because his "examples" of welfare queens drew on existing stereotypes of welfare cheats and resonated with news stories about welfare fraud, they did indeed gain real traction.

Thus, despite the fact that very few cases of individuals engaged in significant welfare fraud have been arrested or tried, as Douglas and Michaels (2004) report, polls from the period show that Americans, in part because of sensationalized welfare cheat language and frequent stories about welfare fraud in the media, vastly overestimated the actual incidence of welfare fraud (which pales by comparison with the level of white-collar fraud committed by wealthy individuals). Some polls found that respondents believed that 40 percent of those on welfare were cheaters although the Department of Health and Human Services estimated at the time that less than 4 percent of individuals receiving welfare actually lied about their financial situation on their applications.

In fact, even during Reagan's presidency the stereotype of the welfare queen was a straw dog. Having more children did not mean receiving more welfare assistance. The actual average welfare increase for having a child was about $60 per month. In some states, women with a newborn did not qualify for any additional aid after her second child was born. In other states, only a small increase was allowed. Having more children simply to get more welfare money would have been a form a self-destructive economics.

Still the stereotype caught hold and many others contributed to and enhanced making this falsehood one of the hardiest chestnuts of contemporary political discourse. In the words of David Zucchino, a Pulitzer Prize-winning reporter, and author of *The Myth of the Welfare Queen* (1999), the notion of the welfare queen is "thoroughly embedded in American folklore."

Adds Kaaryn Gustason (2012), author of "Cheating Welfare: Public Assistance and the Criminalization of Poverty," "It's one of those persistent symbols that come up every election cycle."

For example, Mississippi Governor Haley Barbour, who worked for Reagan as director of the White House Office of Political Affairs in 1985–1986,

THE SOCIAL CONSTRUCTION OF DRUG CONSUMERS ✳ 29

maintained (Kessler 2011) that there was a need to increase co-payments for Medicaid because: "We have people pull up at the pharmacy window in a BMW and say they can't afford their co-payment." Mississippi, in fact, provides one of the lowest levels of Medicaid benefits to working adults in the country. For unemployed parents to qualify, their yearly family income must be less than 24 percent of the poverty level. Working parents can qualify only if they make no more than 44 percent of the federal poverty line. Pregnant women are eligible with income up to 185 percent of the poverty level. This means that a working couple in Mississippi with one child may earn no more than $8,150 a year to qualify for Medicaid, and seniors or pregnant women can earn no more than $20,000 a year. At these levels, people in Mississippi receiving Medicaid who drive a BMW are likely to be very rare, of the sort that birdwatchers call a "mega," one you may never see in your lifetime. Indeed, it is not unreasonable that a family of three earning less than $8,150 annually would have trouble having money for a co-pay, or for much else for that matter. Washington Post fact checker Glenn Kessler (2011) concludes:

> Given that you have to be rather poor to get on Medicaid in Mississippi, it seems highly unlikely the state has many Medicaid recipients driving around BMWs, even used ones. Note that Barbour said "we have people"—suggesting this is not a rare event. The failure of Barbour's aides to provide any documentation for this claim is rather suspicious.

Similarly, during the 2012 presidential race, candidate Rick Santorum, while campaigning in Iowa, said "I don't want to make black people's lives better by giving them somebody else's money," although he later claimed he did not mean to say "black people." During the same campaign, Mitt Romney repeatedly asserted that his opponent, President Obama, wanted to transform America into an "entitlement society." Another candidate, Newt Gingrich, called Obama a food-stamp president, while questioning poor children's work ethic, and saying that poor people should want paychecks, not handouts (Blake 2012). Calling child labor laws "truly stupid," Gingrich told an Iowa audience during the 2012 presidential campaign that children in poor neighborhoods have "no habits of working" nor getting paid for their endeavors "unless it's illegal." Such children, he maintained should be allowed to work as janitors in their schools to earn money and develop a connection to the school (Huisenga 2011).

Franklin Gilliam (1999) of the University of California, Los Angeles became interested in the welfare queen narrative and initiated an interesting study to unravel its effects. An assumption he made in developing the study was that the idea of the welfare queen had gained the status of common knowledge, or what is known in social psychology as a "narrative script." Such scripts distill information and concentrate it in catchwords allowing for the rapid communication of more complex ideas. The welfare queen script Gilliam found consisted of two key components: welfare recipients are disproportionately women (although the largest single group "on welfare" is actually children), and women on welfare are disproportionately African American (even though African Americans comprise only about one tenth of the total number of welfare recipients). In the study, participants watched one of four television stories about the impact of welfare reform on a woman the researchers named Rhonda Germaine. In the story Rhonda worries about the impact of the new welfare laws on her ability to care for her children. A still picture of Rhonda appears at two points in the story; each time it appears, it remains on the screen for about five seconds. Viewers were randomly assigned to one of four groups. Group one watched the news story with Rhonda cast as a white woman. Group two viewed the same story with Rhonda depicted as an African American woman. Group three watched the welfare story without seeing any visual representation of Rhonda. The last group was a control group that did not watch any TV news broadcast about welfare. The researchers inserted a new story about welfare into the middle position of their telecast following the first commercial break. They described the segment as having been selected at random from a news program broadcast during the past week. They found that among white study participants exposure to these script elements reduced their support for welfare programs, increased stereotyping of African Americans, and heightened support for maintaining traditional, unequal gender roles.

Research like this suggests that the media are important, if subtle, sources of popular stereotypes about people on welfare. One extensive content analysis of stories about welfare in news magazines and on network television carried out by Princeton political scientist Martin Gilens (1999) for the 1960s through 1992 found the following:

- Sixty-two percent of stories about poverty that appeared in *TIME*, *Newsweek*, and *U.S. News and World Report* featured African-Americans
- Sixty-five percent of network television news stories about welfare focused on African-Americans
- Fewer African-Americans are portrayed in "sympathetic" stories about poverty and welfare than whites
- News magazines suggest that almost 100 percent of the American underclass as African-Americans.

Based on his analysis, Gilens concluded that negative feelings about welfare among white Americans are rooted in the perception that welfare is a program for African Americans, which in turn, stems from the misrepresentation in the media that most welfare recipients are African Americans and the undeserving poor. Notably, Gilens analysis found that reports in the media about deserving poor focus on the elderly and the working poor who typically are portrayed as poor white individuals whereas poor blacks generally appear in stories about welfare abuse or the perennial underclass.

In the social environment created by such depictions of the ethnic minorities, the poor and welfare, and after what David Rozen (2007:40) has dubbed "a national discourse of extreme vitriol and hyperbole directed at all single, poor mothers, but with a coded sub-text denoting African-American and Latino women," a new law was passed called the Personal Responsibility and Work Opportunity Reconciliation Act (PRWORA). Women no longer were allowed to stay on welfare indefinitely. Additionally, Aid to Families with Dependent Children (AFDC), the needs-based welfare support that disproportionately served ethnic minorities (at least after the 1960s and the Civil Rights Movement) and women was eliminated and replaced with the Temporary Aid to Needy Family program (TANF). As contrasted with AFDC, TANF set a lifetime limit of receivable support of five years. As Nathan and Gais (1998:7) indicated, passage of TANF involved a shift from income assistance to address the survival needs of poor children, to a "service and sanctioning strategy for behavior change" of their mothers. The passage of TANF as well as other constraints on the provision of welfare have been described as components of a "national revival movement calling for the restoration of moral compulsion to the lives of the poor" (Piven and Cloward 2003:135). Of note, TANF became law under a Democratic president, suggesting that the issue is not just conservative strains in the Republican Party but is embedded in a deep layer of social consciousness.

Despite the draconian changes noted above, the term welfare continues to claim a place in the American dialogue on poverty. In his aforementioned article, Liebling (1947) identified the underlying theme of all undeserving-poor narratives: "that the poor are poor because of their sins and whatever they get is too good for them." A parallel narrative, no doubt warmly embraced by most if not all of those who attended Romney's 47 percent speech fund-raiser, is that the rich are rich because of their inherent virtues and contribution to society and whatever they have, no matter how wealthy they are, is wholly deserved (and, further, that concentrating wealth and economic power in their hands will allow it to trickle down and benefit the poor). As the economic and social divide between the very wealthy (the 1 percenters in the contemporary lexicon) and everyone else continues to widen—e.g., the average net worth of the 400 wealthiest people in the United States jumped from $3.8 billion to $4.2 billion in 2011 compared to a 1.5 percent drop in median household income in the country—suggesting the failure of trickle-down economics, the very wealthy have been pressed to amp up the volume on this second narrative. In an interesting comparison of drug users and the superrich, journalist and commentator Lynn Stuart Parramore (2012) observed,

> Like a drug addict turning every cushion upside-down in search of lost change, the 1 percenters are scrounging up every timeworn myth, lame justification and absurd rationalization they can think of to convince us that the rich are super-smart, hard-working job creators instead of greedy parasites refusing to pay their share in taxes and play by the same rulebook as everyone else.

Notably, the changes in welfare policy that forced thousands of women off of government assistance were not successful in eliminating poverty. People leaving welfare for work in the shadow of changes in welfare laws were found generally to earn about $6 an hour or approximately $1,000 a month for a 40 hour work week. Most of the jobs they found did not include insurance benefits (Tepperman 1998). As *Welfare to Work: What Have We Learned* (Joyce Foundation 2002), a study of research on welfare reform in the Midwest, reported, the effects on "poverty reduction have been modest or in some cases disappointing." Most families coming off welfare who rely on wages alone remain poor, where poverty is defined as a yearly income of $$15,510 for a mother with one child and $19,530 for a family of three (2013 figures). Thus they joined the ranks of the working poor, the very group to be attacked by Romney for not paying income tax (because they do not earn enough to pay it according to federal law).

DRUG USERS AS UNWORTHY BEINGS

Embedded in the perspective that many if not most welfare recipients are cheaters is the idea that many also are drug users. This assumed unfailing connection is seen in efforts in numerous states to adopt laws that would require public welfare recipients to take drug tests before receiving any benefits. Movement toward limiting or banning eligibility for welfare among individuals convicted of drug-related crimes (including both distribution and use) began with passage of the 1996 "Gramm Amendment," which imposed a lifetime bar on access to both Food Stamps and TANF. States were granted considerable discretion to modify or cancel the TANF ban. Within public housing, Housing and Urban Development-defined "one strike and you're out" rules allowing for rapid eviction of tenants involved in drug-related crimes or even involvement in drug use by a guest or visitor. Typically, as seen in the subsequent policy adopted in the fall of 2000 by the Anytown Housing Authority (2000), a low standard of proof of drug-involvement became normative: "In order to evict or terminate assistance, a criminal conviction or arrest is not necessary and the AHA need not meet the criminal standard of 'proof beyond a reasonable doubt.'" Within six months of the implementation of this harsh, no second-chance policy, almost 4,000 people had been evicted (and permanently banned) from housing projects around the country. Additionally, Section 902 of welfare reform legislation authorized states to use chemical testing to screen new TANF applicants or to detect illicit drug use otherwise.

Arizona was the first state to impose a testing program. Beginning in 2009, all new welfare recipients were required to undergo a drug test if there was a "reasonable cause" to suspect illicit drug use. To determine reasonable cause, the state asked new recipients whether they had used drugs in the past 30 days, and only those who answered yes were tested. With no penalty for lying, a couple of dozen applicants said they had used drugs. By 2012, 87,000 people had been subjected to the program. How many of these tested positive for drug use? Only one, a factor that has probably limited the enthusiasm in many legislatures for passing such bills (*USA Today* 2012). But the effort goes on. In Colorado, state Representative Jerry Sonnenberg sponsored a similar bill that would require applicants for his state's TANF program to pay for and pass a drug test before receiving government aid. According to Sonnenberg (Alcindor 2012), "If you have enough money to be able to buy drugs, then you don't need the public assistance. I don't want tax dollars spent on drugs." Those who pass the test would be reimbursed for the $8 to $12 cost, but those who fail could not get assistance unless they pass a clean test. Florida passed similar legislation in 2011, an act that the American Civil Liberties Union (ACLU) sees as a presumption of guilt until proven innocent. According to Jason Williamson, an attorney for the ACLU's Criminal Law Reform Project, such laws unfairly stigmatize people and inaccurately imply that people on welfare are more likely to use drugs than other people. In Williamson's view, "This exemplifies the extent to which folks are willing to scapegoat poor people when it suits political interests" (Alcindor 2012). In other states, lawmakers have proposed legislation to implement mandatory drug abuse counseling for people receiving housing assistance (irrespective of their drug use status). Moreover, two states, Ohio and Tennessee have seen bills proposed that would restrict or eliminate welfare eligibility for anyone ever convicted of drug-related felonies (including possession of a small amount of marihuana).

A *USA Today* (2012) editorial based on pending drug use and welfare legislation, however, reviewed the evidence and drew the conclusion that programs to drug-test applicants and recipients of welfare benefits are not useful. In places where such programs have been enacted, few people test positive. As a result, involved states save very little money compared to the upfront costs of implementing testing programs. Moreover, the *USA Today* editorial asserted, these programs perpetuate the inaccurate idea that poor people use drugs more than others and single them out for unconstitutional privacy violations.

Beyond the realm of AFDC/TANF, policy changes have limited the ability of drug users to obtain federal disability payments for drug-related ailments. In 1996, over 200,000 individuals who received SSI or SSDI payments based upon diagnoses of drug and alcohol addiction were removed from recipient rolls because either drug addiction or alcoholism were factors in their determination of disability (Davies et al. 2000). Between December 1996 and January 1997, another 100,000 recipients were removed from the disability assistance rosters because of drug issues (Swartz et al. 2000). Drug problems for these individuals were not defined as real or legitimate medical problems despite the existence of a medical definition of addiction and the subsequent embrace, as discussed in Chapter 6, by the National Institute on Drug Abuse of a view of drug addiction as a relapsing brain disease. Seen as being personally responsible for their disabilities, drug users came to be thought of as unworthy of government supported disability support.

WHEN POVERTY EQUALS DRUG ABUSE

A critical question at stake in this discussion is why is it presumed that the poor are more likely to be involved in drug abuse than other social classes? In part, the linking together of the poor and drug use is perpetuated by regular media images that show drug sales and drug use arrests in poorer neighborhoods. Without question street drug sales are more visible in poor neighborhoods than in those housing other socioeconomic classes. The middle classes and certainly the wealthy can hide their illicit behaviors behind locked doors, on quiet streets, or even behind gated and guarded islands of seeming normalcy. This concealment of drug use is less possible in overcrowded areas with deteriorating infrastructure, homelessness, and intense police presence. Further, poorer neighborhoods have long been allowed to be centers of drug distribution and other illegal activities by the police and larger criminal justice system, despite episodic enforcement in the form of drug or other raids.

Nonetheless, various studies indicate that drug use itself is equally distributed across poor, middle class, and wealthy communities (e.g., Saxe, et al. 2001). Chen, and co-workers (2003), for example, found that alcohol consumption, which is no less drug use than the injection of heroin or the use of methamphetamines, is significantly higher among upper middle class white high school students than among poor black high school students. Their finding underscores a history of research showing that alcohol abuse is much more common among the wealthy than among poor people (Diala, et al. 2004; Galea et al., 2007; Burston and Roberson-Saunders 1995). That the association of drug abuse with poor, minority communities is a misperception is further suggested by research showing higher use rates of use among affluent, suburban, or white youth than among low-income, non-white, urban youth (Luthar and D'Avanzo 1999)

What is of particular note here is not the radical differences in the drug use of the poor and the affluent but the disparities in the consequences of this behavior. While wealthy people use illicit drugs and suffer addiction, and—often, because they receive some form of public scrutiny (e.g., because they are celebrities or relatives of politicians) —are caught breaking drug laws, rarely are they punished to the extent that poor drug users are punished. Notes Paul Wright (2012):

> The unspoken reality is that in America today there exist two systems of criminal justice. One for the wealthy, which includes kid-glove investigations, lackluster prosecutions, drug treatment, light sentences and easy, if any, prison time. The other, for the poor, is one of paramilitary policing, aggressive prosecution, harsh mandatory sentences and hard time.

One notable source of evidence in support of Wright's argument is seen in the comparatively mild sentences given to the children of wealthy politicians when they are caught breaking drug laws. Jenna and Barbara Bush, twin daughters of George W. Bush, for example, were caught (in Jenna's case, two times) by police buying alcohol under age. Their punishment involved several hours of community service, a brief probation, and mandatory enrollment in an alcohol awareness class. The charges were eventually expunged from the Bush daughters' records. A more striking case involves the son of former 30-year Republican Congressman Dan Burton of Indiana, who was on record calling for the death penalty for drug dealers. In 1994 Burton's son, Dan Burton II, was arrested in Louisiana while transporting eight pounds of marihuana from Texas to Indiana. Released on bail, he was arrested again five months later for growing marihuana in his Indianapolis apartment and possessing a shotgun to guard his plants. Despite these serious drug charges, and federal law calling for a mandatory minimum of five years for possessing a firearm during a drug offense, he never faced federal prosecution. He was prosecuted on state charges, and found guilty but his punishment consisted of house arrest, probation, and community service. Similar leniency, the kind rarely seen when the children of poor families are charged with violations of drug laws, occurred following the drug-related arrests of Randall Cunningham, son of anti-drug warrior Congressman Duke Cunningham of California; Richard Riley, Jr., son of Education Secretary Richard Riley; John Murtha, son of Congressman John Murtha; and numerous other children of high office holders. During the period of arrest of these well-linked individuals the average sentence for "low-level" drug-trafficking offenders, was 70.5 months (of which a prisoner typically served about five years) (Bovard 1999). A particularly noteworthy case in this regard involved Cindy McCain, the wife of Senator John McCain of Arizona and daughter of wealthy beer distributor Jim Hensley. Following back surgery, Cindy McCain became addicted to pain-killing drugs. Following investigation by the Drug Enforcement Administration, she admitted to stealing Percocet and Vicodin, schedule 2 narcotic drugs, from the American Voluntary Medical Team, a nonprofit organization she started to deliver medical relief to disaster-stricken or war-torn third-world areas (and which was shut down as a result her theft of drugs from it). Rather than face prosecution and a prison term, which would be standard for a poor person caught committing a similar crime, she was allowed to enter into a pretrial diversion program and avoided acquiring a felony record. Concludes Bovard (2008), "If a poor black woman from Anacostia had committed the crimes that Cindy McCain committed, the black woman might have been sent to prison for the duration of her life."

As the McCain case suggests, even heavily publicized cases of drug use among the affluent never have any sustained impact on the public image of the wealthy as a social class or even on the individuals involved. Moreover, drug treatment, not a prison cell, is the most common social response to drug abuse among individuals from the wealthier social classes. In the media, drug abuse among well-do-do individuals is portrayed as an expression of personal misjudgment, a temporary character defect, or a bad experience rather than as an expression of a lack of social worth. Furthermore, the type of drug treatment that is available to wealthy drug users is very different from the forms of therapy available to poorer drug users enrolled in under-funded, short-term, and narrowly focused programs. Even slots in these kinds of program are often only available to the poor if they can endure long waiting lists, personal indignities, cultural insensitivities, and judgmental providers as well as other insults of the lack of full commitment by society to actually treating the poor effectively for drug dependency and addiction (as opposed to helping them get their drug use under control and back to a more manageable level). Wealthy individuals and their families can afford to pay for the kind of elite treatment programs that, quite literally, only money can buy, namely, programs that fully address the significant and complex psychosocial challenges that both contribute to and are a consequence of prolonged drug use. For example, a 30-day inpatient stay at the world-renowned Betty Ford Center for alcohol and drug treatment located on a 30-acre campus in the resort city of Rancho Mirage, California, costs $32,000. Even more exclusive is Passages Malibu, dubbed by Forbes magazine as one of the most luxurious rehab centers in the world. In 2011, the cost for a month of residential therapy was $88,500.

At the other end of the social hierarchy, assertions about disproportionate drug use among welfare recipients have proved to be questionable. Pollack and co-workers (2001), for example, analyzed nationally representative cross-sectional data, as well as longitudinal Michigan data, to determine the prevalence of drug use among individuals receiving welfare. They found that alcohol dependence was more common among welfare recipients than among people who were not receiving welfare, but, the difference between the two groups was not statistically significant. Additionally, they found that while illicit drug dependence among TANF recipients was more than double the rate among non-recipients, only a small minority of TANF recipients were drug dependent. Pollack et al. (2001) also examined the prevalence of drug use and dependence among TANF respondents in the first three waves of the Women's Employment Study, a panel study of single mothers receiving TANF living in an urban Michigan county. Consistent with other epidemiological findings, illicit drug dependence was rare among all WES respondents (at just over 3 percent), including those still receiving cash assistance.

DRUGS AND MOTHERHOOD

Another side to the intersection of class, race, and gender is seen in dominant social portrayal of drug-using pregnant women and mothers. One consequence of the so-called welfare reform that drastically cut access for poor women to financial and other support is that they were "forced to find alternative resources and to construct survival strategies" (Murphy and Sales 2001). Research by Murphy and Sales with pregnant low-income drug-using women in the San Francisco area examined these strategies, one of which was involvement with drugs. According to Murphy and Sales (2001), the women they interviewed reported that

> [D]rug use helped them overcome some of the adversities in their daily lives. It was sometimes a source of income and usually a source of solace and recreation. Although drug use helped interviewees survive on a day-to-day basis, in the long term, women faced severe consequences.

In part, those consequences were the result of the symbolic targeting of pregnant women involved in drug use as part of the War on Drugs. This targeting, which included the use of "pernicious images of drug-using mothers having babies for the sole purpose of qualifying for government handouts in order to buy drugs and then neglecting and abusing these children" were promulgated by the mass media and by politicians (Campbell 2000; Humphries 1999). In this way, argued Murphy and Sales (2001), "drug users have played a very important role in defining women's and children's poverty as an individual behavioral problem rather than the result of systematic, structural economic inequities." Indeed, drug users often have proven useful in such reassignment of blame from the factors or groups that perpetuate social and economic inequality on to a highly vulnerable population, the poor.

One expression of this use of drug-involved pregnant women was the national outcry in response to the appearance of so-called "crack babies" (babies exposed in utero to crack cocaine) that emerged in the late 1980s (Reinarman and Levine 1989). Observed Murphy and Sales (2001):

> The image of poor inner city African-Americans whose mothering instincts had been destroyed by crack was highly publicized and widely accepted.... Numerous media stories reported that the coming generation would comprise untold numbers of permanently impaired crack babies. It was predicted these impaired infants would topple the

health care delivery and educational systems due to their expensive and lifelong problems. During the same time period, however, there was no comparable public discourse concerning the likelihood of huge expenditures of public resources for a much larger group of problematic infants, tobacco babies, despite considerable available scientific evidence documenting the serious implications for the unborn of maternal tobacco smoking.

In this campaign of image construction, crack-involved pregnant women and mothers were blamed for the creation of permanently impaired children who would not only suffer their whole lives for their mothers' immoral and criminal behavior but would be an economic burden on society. Based on the

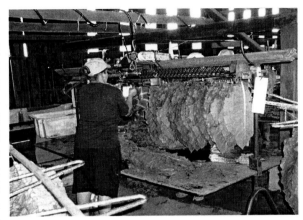

Tobacco drying, Connecticut (Photo by Claudia Santelices)

resulting campaign of moral outrage, articulated through an onslaught of negative media depictions that Jackson (1998) characterized as "an astonishing spree of sloppy, alarmist reporting and racial and economic scapegoating," pregnant women and mothers were arrested, imprisoned, and sentenced to treatment and often lost custody of their children (Humphries et al. 1992). In support of such actions, in 1994, the television news-event program *60 Minutes* aired a segment called "Cracking Down" which acclaimed the success and effectiveness of a South Carolina law under which women who used cocaine while pregnant were arrested and prosecuted under child-abuse statutes. The segment featured scenes of sickly, crack-exposed babies in an intensive-care unit while a nurse pronounced the chances of the children surviving being "real slim" (Jackson 1998). Less evident from the program was that almost all women prosecuted under the statute were African American. Completely invisible in the program was that the nurse who expressed disdainful views of crack-involved mothers later testified that she strongly opposed interracial marriage.

Typical of the images used to depict the irresponsibility and selfish nature of crack-involved women is the following excerpt (Besharov 1989:1) from a story that appeared under the title "Crack Babies: The Worst Threat Is Mom Herself" in the *Washington Post* on August 6, 1989:

> Last week in this city, Greater Southeast Community Hospital released a 7-week-old baby to her homeless, drug-addicted mother even though the child was at severe risk of pulmonary arrest. The hospital's explanation: 'Because [the mother] demanded that the baby be released.' ... Cases like these lead to proposals to expand treatment services for crack-addicted mothers. But at least for now, such services would probably make little difference. Crack addicts typically show little or no interest in prenatal care and are unlikely to seek it until very late in their pregnancy, if ever. Often they present themselves at the hospital only in time to give birth. Some new mothers abandon their sick babies in the hospital—not returning, even if the infant dies, to help bury it.

Headlines and newspaper article titles from the period told the story: "For Pregnant Addict, Crack Comes First" (*Washington Post,* 12/18/89), "Crack's Tiniest, Costliest Victims" (*New York Times,* 8/7/89), "Crack Babies Born to Life of Suffering" (*USA Today,* 6/8/89), "A Time Bomb in Cocaine Babies" (*Washington Post,* 9/18/90), "Parents Who Can't Say 'No' Are Creating a Generation of Misery" (*Los Angeles Times,* 9/21/89), "Disaster in Making: Crack Babies Start to Grow Up" (*St Louis Post-dispatch,* 9/18/90), "Drug Babies Invade Schools" (*San Diego Union-Tribune,* 2/2/92). Crack-involved mothers were accused of birthing a biological underclass of emotionally damaged and misfit children who would become a generation of super-predators at war with a vulnerable society. John Silber, who at the time was president of Boston University, worried aloud that "crack babies ... won't ever achieve the intellectual development to have consciousness of God." Conservative political analyst Charles Krauthammer claimed in his *Washington Post* column: "The inner-city crack epidemic is now giving birth to the newest horror: a bio-underclass, a generation of physically damaged cocaine babies whose biological inferiority is stamped at birth.... Theirs will be a life of certain suffering, of probable deviance, of permanent inferiority." To this, Krauthammer added that "crack babies" would comprise "a race of (sub)human drones" (reported in Vargas 2010). In this way, the 'crack baby' story, coming on the heels of the welfare queen story helped to cement a vision in the popular imagination of the dangerous drug using (usually

African American) woman selling her children's food stamps to finance her abhorrent crack addiction.

Years later, in 2010, after the 'crack baby' scare had faded from the headlines, the *Washington Post* ran a story, that noted "in the two decades that have passed since crack dominated the nation's drug markets, these babies have grown into young adults who can tell their stories, and for the most part, they are tales of success" (Vargas 2010). In fact, no specific disorders or health conditions were ever found among people whose mothers used cocaine while pregnant. Moreover, the crime surge that had been predicted failed to materialize. Rather, by 2008, the national violent crime rate fell to its lowest level since 1972, when the Bureau of Justice Statistics began keeping records. According to FBI data for the District of Columbia, a center of the national crack epidemic and a place early said to be jam-packed with crack using women, from 1990 to 2008, the number of murders per year dropped from 472 to 186, the number of reported rapes fell from 303 to 186, and the number of robberies went from 7,365 to 4,154 (Vargas 2010).

It now is clear that the relationship between maternal crack smoking and adverse child outcomes is complex and affected by many factors (Bandstra et al. 2001). Poverty and lack of prenatal care, it appears, were significant contributing factors in the development of symptoms initially attributed to maternal crack-smoking (Mozes 1999). But, as Murphy and Sales (2001) accentuated, "There are ideological explanations for why these infants continued to be labeled crack babies rather than, in light of scientific findings, poverty babies. In an era of fiscal retrenchment, the notion of poverty babies might engender public sympathy and interfere with the conservative drive to demolish social welfare programs." Despite rising evidence that the "crack baby" story was really about the plight of poor babies and the growing evidence that the depiction of babies exposed to crack and women using crack were based on discredited assertions, in 1998 *60 Minutes* re-aired its "Cracking Down" without correcting any of the misinformation it contained, further perpetuating the apparently very useful "crack baby" myth.

THE GREATER SIN OF FEMALE DRUG USE

While both men and women abuse drugs, the experience and effects of drug abuse are not gender neutral nor are the meanings society attaches to drug use by women the same as those constructed for men. Moreover, because of differences in the gendered life experiences of women and men and the ways gender relations order social life and social institutions, drug use is not quite the same thing across gender. There are, in other words, drawing from Daly (1998), what might be called "gendered pathways to drug abuse." Most importantly, drug use patterns reflect the underlying cultural construction of male superiority and male social and political-economic domination over women (Miller and Mullins 2009).

Research indicates that female drug abusers are more likely than their male counterparts to have a history of physical and/or sexual abuse or emotional trauma, with as many as 70% of women in drug treatment reporting histories of such mistreatment (Najavits et al. 1997). As Chesney-Lind and Pasko (2004:5) indicate, the earlier victimization of girls compared to boys, "set[s] the stage for their entry into youth homelessness, unemployment, drug use, survival sex (and sometimes prostitution), and ultimately, other serious criminal acts." Women, in fact, are more likely to begin abusing drugs or alcohol after a specific traumatic life experience (Najavits, 2002; Nelson-Zlupko et al, 1995; Virginia Department of Mental Health, Mental Retardation and Substance Abuse Services 2004). From a feminist perspective, these patterns suggest the many ways that drug abuse among women is a product of varied forms of male dominance and the physical and emotional abuse that find impact across women's experience in society. Drug abuse among women, from this perspective, can be seen as being closely tied to the strategies women use to navigate gender-stratified social environments. As Bepko (1991:1) maintains, drug abuse among women involves "a process in which individuals make dysfunctional attempts to have control over their own experience within a relational context.... [Thus] addiction is a microcosmic process that reflects and is perhaps a metaphor for imbalances of power in the larger social arena." Beyond gender differences in the emergence and expressions of drug abuse, are notable contrasts in consequences. These contrasts mirror the ways gender influences society's tolerance of drug use and the intensified social stigmas suffered by female drug abusers (Kauffman et al. 1997).

Generally, because of androcentric bias, drug-dependent women are socially perceived as having more significant personal problems, as being in greater violation of societal norms, and as being more deviant than male drug users. The added violation of female drug users involves their transgression of what are held to be critical social standards involving being a "good woman." The major concern is that the female addict fails to fulfill her vital social responsibility to be a nurturer and caretaker and is deemed as a result not only irresponsible but reprehensible (Hodgins et al. 1997; Manhal-Baugus, 1998). Women of color are especially stigmatized in this regard (Brissett-Chapman

1998), as gender, race, and class are intimately interconnected axes of social domination and inequality (Anderson and Collins 2012).

Even on the streets, in the underground drug economy, women are disadvantaged. As Maher (1997) has shown in her ethnographic account of the illicit street drug trade, there exists a gendered division of labor in income generating activities (also see Ripoll et al. 2002, Singer et al. 2013). Maher (1997:54) documents the ways women are "clearly disadvantaged compared to their male counterparts" but stresses the need for striking a balance between

> the twin discourses of victimization and volition that inform current understandings of women's drug-related lawbreaking. While this space must be large enough to include the constraints of sexism, racism, and poverty that [structure] women's lives, it cannot be so big as to overwhelm the active, creative and often contradictory choices, adaptations and resistances that constitute women's criminal activities (Maher 1997:201).

Another consequence of the stigmas borne by women that have been described in the drug-abuse research literature is the bias against female clients by treatment professionals. Research shows that treatment providers are more likely to describe the female drug-abusing clients as difficult, less compliant, and less responsive to treatment. Reviews of the literature reveal that many healthcare professionals hold especially denigrating stereotypical views and negative attitudes toward women who use illicit drugs (McLaughlin and Long 1996). Additionally, given their experience of gendered societal expectations, woman drug users are more likely to experience higher levels of guilt and shame in acknowledging their drug dependency than do men. Moreover, drug use treatment traditionally has been informed by male experience and from a male perspective (Walitzer and Sher 1996). These patterns are reflected in feminist analyses of abusive drinking among women and the early response of Alcoholics Anonymous

> The social stigma, shame, and taboo of being a female alcoholic was so great that many women felt too inhibited to admit their alcoholism. It was thought that "nice" women didn't become drunks ... and the cultural image of the "moral woman" ... was not easily extinguished by men or women inside AA, even though most AA members believed alcoholism was a physiological disease and not a problem of character.

Moreover, as women began to share their stories inside AA, they perceived a double standard applied to them as alcoholic women. Also, some of the men and some of the wives of the alcoholics felt it was dangerous to include women in AA groups, where indiscrete relationships might develop (Sanders 2009:8).

It is consequently not surprising to discover that women have not done as well in drug-abuse treatment as men, with rates of entry into treatment, retention, and completion of treatment being lower for women than for men (Hodgins et al. 1997). Feminists have critiqued the self-centeredness embedded in the AA model of treatment, which has spread as well to the treatment of other forms of chemical abuse and has been adopted in many drug treatment programs. Feminist critics argue, the underlying culture of the twelve-step movement is not gender neutral but rather is ultimately detrimental to women, in that it encourages women to see themselves as the problem rather than recognizing the social origins of their suffering and organizing to achieve change in the socio-political environment (Rapping 1997).

ARRESTED WHILE BLACK

Of importance in this examination of social stigmatization is the fact that the poor, particularly the African American poor and other ethnic minorities, are arrested and incarcerated at rates that are disproportionate to their levels of drug use (Covington 1997). In a report entitled "Decades of Disparity: Drug Arrests and Race in the United States," issued by Human Rights Watch (HRW) (2009), for example, it is noted that African Americans have been arrested for drug offenses nationwide at higher rates than whites for nearly three decades, even though they engage in drug offenses at comparable rates. Based on FBI data, the HRW report indicates that African Americans were arrested on drug charges at rates that were 2.8 to 5.5 times as high as those of white adults in every year from 1980 through 2007, the last year for which complete data were available. With specific reference to crack cocaine, while studies suggest that about 15 percent of the nation's cocaine users (in both powder and crack forms) are African American, they account for about 90 percent of those convicted on crack cocaine charges (Davidson 1999). Overall, about one in three of the more than 25.4 million adult drug arrestees in recent years was African American, suggesting the extent and persistence of racial disparities in US drug law enforcement. In 2000, for example, the rate of incarceration for African American males nationwide was almost 3,500 per 100,000 people. By comparison, for white males the rate of incarceration was below 500 per 100,000. On average, African American males were almost 8 times more likely to be imprisoned than white males. The racial disparities in incarceration are even more drastic for young African American men between the ages of 18 and 19 years and 25 and 29 years compared to their white counterparts; thus African Americans in these age groups were almost 9 times more likely to be behind bars than whites of the same age (Nunn 2002).

Another measure of the extent of mass incarceration in the African American community is the percentage that is in prison at any given time. In some locations, one third of the adult African American male population always is incarcerated. At the national level, while 1.6 percent of the African American population is in prison, almost 10 percent of African American males ages 25 to 29 years are in prison (Nunn 2002). Overwhelmingly, drug arrests are the source of the mass incarceration of African Americans, but they encompass arrests of other ethnic minority populations as well (Tonry 1996).

State-by-state data show that African Americans were arrested for drug offenses at rates in individual states that were 2 to 11.3 times greater than the rate for whites. Additionally, the report reveals that arrests for drug possession have greatly exceeded arrests for the sale of drugs every year since 1980. Moreover, the proportion of drug arrests for possession has been increasing relative to drug sales and has amounted to at least 80 percent of drug arrests annually since 1999 (Human Rights Watch 2009). As a result, there are over one million African American children with an incarcerated parent (or about one in nine), and more than half of these imprisoned parents were convicted of a drug or other nonviolent offense (Weston 2010).

THE WAR ON DRUGS AND THE WAR ON THE POOR

The class and racial enforcement of drug laws contributes to a significant social divide in the impact of the enduring War on Drugs (Singer 2004). As Weston (2010), a professor of sociology at Harvard University, emphasizes:

> Drugs are intensively criminalized among the poor but largely unregulated among the rich. The pot, coke and ecstasy that enliven college dorms, soothe the middle-class time bind and ignite the octane of capitalism on Wall Street are unimpeded by the street sweep, the prison cell and the parole-mandated urine tests that are routine in poor neighborhoods.

In this regard, Robert Trojanowicz (1991) while at the National Center for Community Policing, pointed out a pertinent pattern in drug law enforcement:

> In New York City, narcotics officers are regularly assigned to the Port Authority, where they routinely confront bus patrons and ask to search their bags for drugs.... But why do the police target bus passengers (who tend to come from lower socioeconomic classes where minorities are overrepresented)?

At the same time, the health and social consequences of drug abuse are decidedly greater for the poor, who have few resources to spend on drug treatment and less access to quality care. Existing studies show that: 1) social deprivation and marginalization is associated with the most extensive forms of illicit drug user; 2) social and economic deprivation result in less access to health care and drug treatment; and 3) capacity for overcoming drug dependence is lower among the poor, having less access to meaningful social roles and adequate livelihood (Singer 2008). Critical to the impacts of drug use on the poor is marginalization. Thus, in a study over 1,500 active drug injectors from the ALIVE cohort, Genberg et al. (2011) found that residential relocation was associated with greater likelihood of long-term cessation of drug injection, but the impact of residential relocation varied

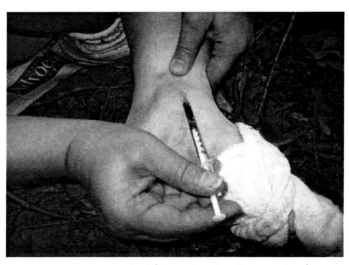

Drug injection in Hartford (Photo by Claudia Santelices)

depending on the deprivation of the drug user's new neighborhood. Moving from a highly deprived to less deprived neighborhood had the greatest positive impact on ending drug injection, while staying in the most deprived neighborhoods was detrimental to people's likelihood of ceasing drug injection. What was critical to continued drug injection in this study was not the mindset, personality, addiction level, world view, value system, or other personal characteristics of drug users, rather it was the nature of the neighborhood in which they lived.

This interpretation is supported by a study in Detroit by Boardman et al. (2001) of the effects of neighborhood disadvantage, experience of stress, and drug use. Using the 1995 Detroit Area Study and tract-level census data, they found that increased social stressors and higher levels of psychological distress among residents of poor neighborhoods is associated with drug use, especially among individuals with the lowest annual incomes. Those with the fewest resources living in the poorest areas are the least likely to be able to "assuage feelings of depression, anxiety and despair [without] drug use, which [for them] may be [the most available] and affordable coping response."

Beyond poverty, chronic exposure to racism and classism is a known stressor (Baer et al. 2013; Kreiger 2005). Singer and colleagues (Baer et al. 2013) have used the term "oppression illness" to characterize such structurally imposed social stress. The psychological effects of this traumatic stress disorder, including depression, anger, and self-blame, are produced by the combined effects of being subject over time to intense social opprobrium (e.g., in the form of racial hatred, sexism, class discrimination) and the internalization of this reproach in the form of self-hatred. Other forms of social misery endured by the poor and ethnic minorities are less visible and more subtle, but consist of daily, structurally imposed insults, indignities, and emotional injuries stemming from the experience of status inequalities. These psychological wounds, which, borrowing from Sennett and Cobb (1972), can be referred to as "hidden injuries of oppression," include both repeated exposure to disrespect (across class, race/ethnicity, sexual identity, and gender lines) and the enduring frustrations of prolonged social failure in the American culture of personal achievement. For example, each time people of color walk into a store and feel that they are being unduly scrutinized by white store employees the resulting feeling of indignity is a hidden injury of oppression. For the inner city poor such experiences, in varied form and social location, are a recurrent component of everyday oppression.

Not only do poor areas with high levels of unemployment and deteriorating infrastructure produce an inordinate level of social stress that may contribute to self-medicating drug use, they often involve a social environment in which involvement in drug sales is an established and easily accessible (perhaps the most accessible) way of earning money. Based on his ethnographic research with young Latinos involved in the drug trade in New York City, Bourgois (2003b:4) asks: "Why should these young men and women take the subway to minimum wage jobs—or even double minimum wage jobs—in downtown offices when they can usually earn more, at least in the short run by selling drugs on the street corner in front of their apartment or school yard? In fact, I am always surprised that so many inner-city men and women remain in the legal economy and work nine to five plus overtime, barely making ends meet."

During the 1980s and 1990s, many inner city areas like the one described by Bourgois experienced an intensification of concentrated poverty due to globalization, the flight of capital and production, and the loss of jobs in urban centers (Singer 2007). As Bourgois notes,

> The economic base of the traditional working class has eroded throughout the country. Greater proportions of the population are being socially marginalized. The restructuring of the world economy by multinational corporations, finance capital, and digital electronic technology, as well as the exhaustion of social demographic models for public sector intervention on behalf of the poor [e.g. the welfare state] have escalated inequalities around class ethnicity and gender" (Bourgois 2003b:319).

The US inner city, a sociocultural and experiential space that Wacquant (2001) has termed the hyperghetto, today functions as a kind of ethno-class prison "in that it encloses a stigmatized population with its own distinctive organizations and culture." This development, a product of technoeconomic and related social changes that began take hold during the 1980s and 1990s (the era of the rise of crack cocaine), reflects a broader societal pattern involving the devaluation of physical labor, continuing shrinkage of working class salaries, and a dramatic loss of working-class jobs. As a consequence of these sweeping structural changes, argues Wacquant, the contemporary inner city has lost many of its earlier communal features and acquired a social structure and cultural climate that parallels those of a prison. For inner city youth, legitimate opportunities for a dignified level of income acquisition have been widely replaced by illicit jobs in the underground drug-fueled opportunity structure. Under these conditions, the ever-vibrant drug trade and its alluring if ephemeral promise of conspicuous wealth for the inner city poor "remains a ready but risky source of casual employment for low-education men and women with no legitimate prospects" (Weston 2010).

Still, despite all of these factors, considering alcohol and illicit drugs together, there is evidence to suggest that wealthy people are at least as likely if not more likely than poor people to be drug abusers. The drug use of wealthy people, however, is less visible to the wider society as it takes place behind closed doors and not, very often, on the street in the view of the public. Consequently, as Saxe et al. (2001b:1987) point out, public intervention programs "focus on visible manifestations of substance use. In particular, in the framework of prevention efforts, programs focus on illicit drug use in poor and minority communities where drug markets are most visible. Yet visibility of drugs in particular communities does not necessarily imply drug use among residents of those communities." The association of drug abuse with poor neighborhoods, these researchers argue, may be a product of the tendency to associate crime and drug use, leading to the assumption that because more street crime occurs in poor, inner city neighborhoods there must be more drug use there. Ethnographic research on the drug scenes in urban neighborhoods, however, reveals that suburban drug users drive into the inner city to purchase drugs (Singer and Mirhej 2004; Williams 1992). Research by Riley (1997) on heroin and cocaine trafficking in six cities, for example, found that Whites were more likely than African Americans to buy drugs outside of their own neighborhoods and to buy them indoors. As a result, visible drug use and sales that occur in a neighborhood may not reflect elevated levels of drug use by people who live in that neighborhood (Ensminger et al. 1997)

The emergence of inner city, generally heavily minority populated, urban areas as centers of drug distribution has a long history. This pattern traces to the large migration of rural African Americans in the South into the cities of the North beginning in the early 1900s in one of the largest population shifts in US history. In huge cities like Chicago—which has been dubbed the most segregated city in America—the new arrivals encountered intense racism, imposed social marginalization, family disruption, routine structural discrimination, and urban poverty (which experientially was more oppressive than the rural poverty most migrants had endured in the South). The great migration of African Americans was fueled by hopes of social and economic advancement and a craving for liberation from the stultifying Southern-style Jim Crow racism. For the most part the migrants were young, single, and optimistic, but the urban environments that received them were anything but warm and welcoming.

As parts of northern cities filled up with African Americans, the dominant white society responded with a collective, if largely unspoken, decision to abandon the areas where the migrants were settling, leaving behind decaying schools, failing utilities and services, and few opportunities for legal employment, thereby condemning the inhabitants to perpetual poverty. During the years of Prohibition, from 1920 to 1933, African American neighborhoods "became the place where whites practiced their vices" (James and Johnson 1996: 16). Black-owned jazz clubs, after-hours clubs, houses of prostitution, gambling halls, dance clubs, and other sites of recreation and illicit behavior emerged as important social centers for the growing African American urban population. Whites, desiring excitement and an escape from the depressing economy, flocked to the inner city "to hear African American music, to party, to patronize houses of prostitution, and to gamble" (James and Johnson 1996:17). As Drake and Cayton (1970) point out, these centers of congregation often became points of contact between the purveyors of pleasure "on the illigit" and their clientele—commercial sex workers, bootleggers, marihuana peddlers, and pimps. These places, they note (Drake and Cayton 1970:610) often were "merely 'fronts' and 'blinds' for the organized underworld.... The primary institutions of the underworld [were] the tougher taverns, the reefer pads, the gambling dens, the liquor joints, and the call houses and buffet-flats where professional prostitutes cater to the trade in an organized fashion."

It was during this era that inner city areas, as marginalized sectors of the city, emerged as drug distribution sites for the wider urban environment. In poor neighborhoods, drug laws may at times be fiercely enforced but unevenly so with visible routine illicit drug sales occurring in key "hot spot" street corners and open-air drug markets or at more dispersed more public or less public sites through neighborhoods. Poor communities, however, commonly have questions about the objectives of street drug-law enforcement:

> The community feels that while there are more drugs sold and used in majority neighborhoods, law enforcement has no interest in those people or those crimes. The real money and the real benefits of the drug trade go to high-level figures outside the community. There is strong feeling that the drug trade could not exist without the acquiescence and support of the government and law enforcement, that the government actually manages the drug trade, and that the CIA invented crack and brought in it into the community. High levels of enforcement, arrest,

and incarceration in minority neighborhoods are seen as a deliberate outside attack, designed as a way to incapacitate strong young minority men and provide work for law enforcement agencies and prison staff (Kennedy and Wong 2009:8).

Various analysts have concluded that the enduring flow of drugs into poor neighborhoods as distribution centers for a wider suburban periphery is facilitated, at least in part, by police corruption. Certainly it is not difficult to find cases of police on the drug take. Smith (2012), for example, maintains a website that provides weekly reports on police (or related criminal justice) drug-corruption cases around the country. For the week of October 31, 2012, for example, he reports cases in Gary, Indiana; Chicago, Illinois; Waveland, Mississippi; and Flomaton, Alabama. The prior week, a former New York City Police Department officer was sentenced to 15 years in prison for selling two stolen guns to a local drug group to pay off his drug debts. The General Accounting Office reports that from 1993 to 1998 the FBI initiated about 400 state and local drug-related police corruption arrests resulting in the conviction of over 300 police officers. More recently, in 2001 eight San Antonio police officers were arrested for plotting to protect a cocaine delivery. During the same period in Los Angeles, the Rampart Scandal came to light as numerous officers in the anti-drug unit were indicted on corruption charges that included drug dealing. Also during this period three police officers in Florida were indicted for drug trafficking, including using their patrol cars to transport drugs for local drug dealers (Drug Policy Alliance 2002).

It is not hard to understand how the drug war breeds police corruption; there are vast sums of money available to drug dealers that can be spent in this way and police may be underpaid and seeking additional income. Allegations of official complicity in the drug trade in US cities, like the one encapsulated in the quote on community attitudes above, have a long history. Most recently this charge has been leveled by Guillermo Terrazas Villanueva, spokesperson for the Chihuahua, Mexico state government. According to Terrazas, "It's like pest control companies, they only control…. If you finish off the pests, you are out of a job. If they finish the drug business, they finish their jobs" (Arsenault 2012). While other Mexican officials dispute this assertion, it is evident from multiple local cases that one factor in the concentration of drug trafficking in poor neighborhoods is police corruption and complicity, as well as cultural attitudes about the poor and ethnic minorities.

CONCLUSION: THE USEFUL THREAT OF
THE BLACK BOGYMAN DRUG USER

The association discussed in this chapter between poverty, ethnic minorities, gender biases and people's conceptions and patterns of drug use, as well as the pejorative sentiments that help to propel stigmatization, contribute to the identification and demonization of the drug user and addict as the ultimate social deviant, the very embodiment of beings that are alien and threatening to the dominant mainstream society. In the minds of middle class and suburban-dwelling Americans and their elected officials from similar or higher class backgrounds, inner city ghettos are "filled with black men mugging whites for money to pay for heroin and then injecting this evil drug so that they can spend the rest of the day nodding away in a blissful vacuum" (Iiyama et al. 1976: 17). So compelling for them is this constructed image, despite being so loaded with inaccuracies as revealed by social scientific research, that it has helped drive continued media accounts, the enactment of drug-related laws and policies, the incarceration of massive numbers of individuals, the withdrawal of the social safety net for the poor, and the disruption of minority communities. Feeding this perilous image are angered attitudes about African American women as breeders of children as part of an indolent scam to swindle the hard-working taxpayer into supporting their unproductive yet lavish lifestyles, and about the male children of these women, exposed to drugs in utero or soon afterward, who routinely become worthless, drug-crazed, and violent threats lurking at the gates of innocent morally correct and primarily white neighborhoods. While disputable at every turn, these images do not easily go away, and they are not subject to refutation through a presentation of mere facts. This is the case because they are useful images, they serve important social functions for those who embrace them, including justifying discriminatory laws and social practices that sustain an unlevel playing field that works to the advantage of wealthier sectors of society at grave cost to poorer sectors.

CHAPTER TWO

Drug Users through the Ages
When Did We Decide Addicts Were a Separate Category?

E xactly when the Othering of addicts began can be traced to the 18th century, probably to the gin epidemic of London. Prior to our concerted effort to find evidence of the concept of the addict in the writings of the ancients, we had always thought that it had been present since the discovery of intoxicating preparations. We could not, however, find it in any of those writings, from the Ghitas to the Gilgamesh epic, to the Torah, to Plato's *Symposium,* to the letters of Paul the Apostle. All of these sources made mention of strong drink, and most warned against drunkenness, but none attributed drunkenness as a chronic condition. In all of these venerable writings, the lone example of the habitual addict appears in Homer's *Odyssey,* in which Odysseus and his crew encountered and are enticed by the Lotus Eaters, whose lifestyle seemed to reflect an addicted condition. Nevertheless, because the described behaviors resembled no known addictive pattern, involving no known drug, the appearance of the lotus eaters in *The Odyssey* may be a product of an active imagination, or perhaps a story from another source, rather than an expression of personal experience. In order to trace when and where humankind came to "recognize" addicts and addiction, this chapter begins by positing humankind's ability to ingest toxins and derive something other than illness or death from them as a phenomenon with deep evolutionary precedents.

Only speculation, albeit backed by archaeological and ethnographic evidence, is possible with regard to the process of discovering plant-derived preparations that gave pleasure to their users. After laying out the fundamentals of drug use among humans, this chapter proceeds in its search for instances in which writers of ancient texts perceived some of the people they knew or observed as drunkards or addicts. It appears, as noted, that the concept of addiction (including alcoholism) received full articulation in the 19th century, and that articulation co-occurred with the widespread availability of truly concentrated intoxicants, especially alcohol, opioids, and

The Social Value of Drug Addicts: The Uses of the Useless, by Merrill Singer and J. Bryan Page, 53–70.
© 2014 Left Coast Press, Inc. All rights reserved.

cocaine. This chapter's narrative focuses on alcohol, because it has the longest documented history of human consumption. In our pursuit of instances where ancient writers attributed chronicity to the observed use of drugs, we also inspect the evidence on opioids since concentrated preparations made it relatively easy to become intoxicated, thereby increasing the likelihood of intoxication in individual users.

EVOLUTIONARY PRECEDENTS

Millennia before the first archaeologically detectable evidence that humankind consumed some plants or plant products to become intoxicated, humans were interacting with biospheres and discovering by accident the plants or plant-derived preparations that made their senses function differently. McGovern's (2003) research, for example, limits the hard evidence of wine and its use and storage to 7000 or 8000 years before the present. Nevertheless, we can assume that humans were exposed to fermented grapes and other fruit long before that. Likewise, across millennia of interaction with plants, paleolithic humans were likely to have tasted of plants, such as the flowers or fruit of datura, that caused them to have a variety of altered nerve functions, perhaps depressant, perhaps stimulant, perhaps hallucinogenic. The fact that humans willingly repeated these exposures tells us that on some very basic level, the human body was ready to process the toxins in wine and other plant material and then derive some kind of benefit from the plants' effect on the nervous system.

An understanding of how humans have come to use plant-derived drugs and how plants have come to produce drugs has emerged as neurobiology and botanical pharmacology have become increasingly sophisticated at the molecular level. The process of knowledge development began in the mid-1990s with the assertion that the concept of "evolutionary novelty" explained human use of plant-derived drugs (e.g., Nesse and Berrige 1997). Later theorists held that plants and animals constantly develop action-and-reaction features involving plant toxins and defenses against those toxins, leaving humans with some of the same defenses originally developed by herbivores millions of years earlier (e.g., Sullivan et al. 2008).

In the former argument, Nesse and Berrige (1997) excluded human beings, at least temporarily, from the influence of evolutionary process in the human response to psychotropic plants, holding that when humans got around to trying some psychoactive plants, they derived reward messages to the brain that bypassed other systems for processing the total effect of the toxins being ingested. In other words, whatever was negative or not useful in the experience of eating opium or chewing coca was essentially over-shadowed by the reinforcement that went straight to the pleasure centers of the mid-brain (Nesse and Berrige 1997). Consequently, humans liked and wanted this experience again, even though it did not really meet full criteria for being beneficial to the human consumer (e.g., providing nourishment or enhancing performance). Once they had discovered the "empty treat" of the drug high, humans began to seek the reward repeatedly.

The latter argument, forwarded by Sullivan, Hagen, and Hammerstein (2008), rests on the fact that plants and animals have been evolving for millennia at counter-purposes—plants developing aversive toxins to put animals off of eating them and animals developing metabolic mechanisms to filter out the plant-derived toxins so they could keep on eating. The characterization of the cytochrome P450 system, which resides in the human liver, but exists in many other animals as well, has fed this particular theory, because it provides strong evidence of the evolutionary universality of animals' internal mechanisms that counteract the effects of plant toxins. Drug plants present an array of alkaloids that often are toxic in high concentrations, but as they occur in plant material, they are not so toxic as to be intolerable to humans equipped with the cytochrome P450 mitigation system. At least that may be true for some humans, as the accumulated evidence on the workings of cytochrome P450 show considerable variation across human populations (Sullivan et al. 2008) regarding what toxins are metabolized and thoroughly excreted. So, for example, Asian populations may respond to the nearly universal plant-derived toxin alcohol differently from European populations, although most human populations have categorized alcohol in the form of fermented beverages as desirable and often a complement to other food.

The cytochrome P450 system aids in processing plant-derived toxins other than alcohol, helping to keep our omnivorous ancestors out of trouble and mitigating the impact of consuming plants that contain drugs or alcohol produced from plants. If we follow the logic of this particular speculative theory to its conclusion, the eventual elaboration of the human nervous system led to circumstances in which the creatures endowed with a complex brain might discover and derive gratification from plant material that did not necessarily nourish them but did make them feel different. If that feeling was pleasant, these creatures were smart enough to seek out ways to repeat it. Although the original authors of these theories did not engage in this level of description, one could imagine our pre-primate ancestors, for example, foraging for leafy vegetables and coming upon a succulent-looking proto-tobacco that had developed an emetic toxin—nicotine—that it contained in sufficient amounts to put our ancestors off by making them nauseous. Some of these ancestors, however, acquired by mutation or other genetic process a modification that enabled them to process modest amounts of nicotine without getting sick, and that allowed continued consumption of the proto-tobacco, which for some reason—perhaps its ability to revive a tired body—improved their survival chances within the species' total population.

Flash forward millions of years, and we find humans somewhat disengaged from the back-and-forth counter-adaptations suggested by Sullivan, Hagen and Hammerstein (2008), but they are a curious species, constantly discovering new components of nature's bounty and testing for nutritional or other value. As fully developed *Homo sapiens sapiens,* they now have brains that are so elaborately developed that they value far more than whether or not a plant material alleviates hunger and provides nourishment. A human may prize a plant or plant product if it makes him/her feel different—perhaps more energetic or somnolent, or if it alleviates pain. The combination of curiosity, the aptitude to store in their cultural warehouse vast amounts of environmental information, the capacity to appreciate a wide variety of effects associated with consumption, and the physiologic equipment to process safely a wide range of the toxins that may be involved makes the contemporary human being (i.e., anybody born after 20,000 BCE) the ideal explorer of plants and what they have to offer. These features of humanity also made it inevitable that the vast majority would discover something in their local environments to alter their consciousness and incorporate into cultural traditions. And this is precisely what occurred in global history.

Left out of this anthropocentric explanation is recognition that what appears to be nonhuman animal consumption of plants that contribute to what appear to be altered physiological states and states of consciousness (Huffman 2003). It is well known, for example, that cats are highly attracted to the valerian plant (*Valeriana officinalis*) and catnip (*Nepeta cataria*). Sniffing and consuming these plants appears to push cats into a state of observable satisfaction. Similarly, cattle will readily eat plants that contain alkaloids that seem to have a narcotic effect (Dudley 2002). Additionally, birds and various other animals have been observed seeking out and consuming highly fermented fruit and afterward showing signs of being drunk, such as stumbling and acting as if they are noticeably under the influence. All of these behaviors suggest that many species in addition to humans have long evolutionary histories consuming plants with psychoactive properties. In the assessment of ethnopharmacologist Ronald Siegel (2005:10), "ethnological and laboratory studies ... and analyses of social and biological history, suggest that the pursuit of intoxication with drugs is a primary motivational force in the behavior of organisms." Siegel labels this behavior "the fourth drive" in a list that includes the biologically based motivators of hunger, thirst, and sex. As this discussion suggests, human involvement with psychotropic plants builds on and constitutes a set of cultural elaborations of more broadly shared and evolutionarily far older behavioral patterns in diverse species.

HUMANKIND AND INTOXICATION

Wine and its consumption provide good starting points for discussing the beginnings of human intoxication because humankind has a documented continuous history of drinking wine and getting drunk from its effects that spans all of recorded history and reaches back into the realm of oral history that preceded it. This background story of wine and its consumption provides useful material on the formation of ancient peoples' attitudes about intoxication and altered states of consciousness.

Because the receptacles used by Paleolithic hunter-gatherers were likely to be made of organic material, such as animal skin and/or reed basketry, archaeologists hold out little hope of finding conclusive evidence of the very earliest instances of humans' consumption of fermented grapes, or proto-wine, which might easily have occurred over 10,000 years ago, given the climate shifts associated with the recession of the last Ice Age (McGovern 2003: 8). The availability of the fruit, Vitis vinifera sylvestris, that is ancestral to the grapes used in contemporary winemaking occurred in several different sites in what we now call the Middle East. Archaeologists have been able to find apparent wine residues in ancient pottery, pointing to the presence in ancient parts of contemporary Georgia, Turkey, and Iraq of traditions of wine production (McGovern 2003: 40–42) possibly as early as 8,000 years ago, but at least 7,000 years ago.[1]

The presence of this potentially intoxicating and addictive drink, however, did not necessarily lead to the establishment of a sub-population of consumers identified as problematic by the rest of their group. Rather, the ancients expressed a caution about wine's effects when drunk to excess (Grivetti 1995:10). In ancient India, China, and Egypt, physicians and men regarded as wise consistently expressed ambivalent opinions about the consumption of wine. The Ayurvedic physicians of India (ca.1400 BCE) were aware of wine's benefits, attributing, among other things, exhilaration, nourishment, and freedom from fear, grief, or fatigue to its consumption (Grivetti 1995). They also recognized a downside to wine drinking in excess:

One who saturates himself excessively with . . . fresh wine . . . and at the same time abstains from physical movements including day-sleep, suffers from diseases . . . such as diabetic boils, urticarial patches, itching, anemia, fever, leprosy, anorexia, drowsiness, impotency, over-obesity, disorders of consciousness, sleepiness, swelling, and other disorders (Grivetti 1995:10).

Despite the subtext of wine drinking as a chronic condition, however, they did not pathologize excessive drinking to the point of giving this behavior a separate name. That name did not enter the literature on alcohol consumption until the middle of the 19th century, when Magnus Huss wrote about alcoholism (Phillips 2000: 271). During the 3,300 years after the Ayurvedic writers recorded their opinions about wine, philosophers and physicians made various observations about the effect of wine drinking. Egyptians warned against wine's duality, noting that while it made the drinker feel good, its consumption in excess could lead to unacceptable behavior (Grivetti 1995:11). Similarly, Hippocrates noted wine's positive effects, going so far as to include wine in some of his remedies, even what sounds like a wine diet: "It is better to be full of wine than full of food." (Grivetti 1995:12) Nevertheless, he also recognized the potential harm of drinking wine in excess. Throughout the ancients' musings on wine and its influence, a pattern of duality emerges in which wine in moderation is seen as beneficial, and wine in excess is seen as harmful, or at least embarrassing. With the exception of the Ayurvedic physicians, however, the ancients' discussions focused on the acute intoxicating effects of wine, not on the long-term effect of addiction. We should also note that the ancient Egyptians, Greeks, and Romans almost always diluted wine with water, making the task of achieving an intoxicating dose more difficult than if it were consumed neat, or without dilution. Depending on how much water was added to the wine, the resulting drink may have had the rough equivalent of the proportion of alcohol found in beer (4–8 percent by volume).

Were there no people labeled as chronic drunks in the ancient world? If there were, the available literature does not tell us much about them. Perhaps they did not congregate in easily recognizable locales, such as present-day Seattle's Skid Road, New York's Bowery, or Miami's overpasses. Among the Greeks and Romans, in the writings of Plato about the Greek *symposium* and Plutarch and others on the Roman equivalent *convivium* there was a sense that the participants were not drunkards but men who intended to drink on the occasion of one of these gatherings (Standage 2005:78). Still, even in the passages describing people given to excess drink, it appears that the ancient writers focused not on chronicity so much as on the harm that excessive drinking sessions do to the drinker. For example, in Plato's *Symposium*, one participant suggests that after the previous night's excesses the group might adopt a drinking policy:

> ... [T]hey were about to commence drinking, when Pausanias said, "And now, my friends, how can we drink with least injury to ourselves? I can assure you that I feel severely the effect of yesterday's potations, and must have time to recover; and I suspect that most of you are in the same predicament, for you were of the party yesterday. Consider then: How can the drinking be made easiest?" (MIT Classics 2011).

Pausanias wanted not a reprise of the previous night's excesses, but to establish some principles by means of which the same group who were drunk the previous night would drink but avoid excess on the night at hand. Ancient texts repeatedly give the reader the sense that each drunken occasion was to the participants and witnesses more significant than the frequency of these occasions.

Saint Augustine's writings on the subject of drunkenness (cf. Cook 2006:52–56) indicate that early Christian philosophy regarding intoxication with alcoholic beverages deplored drunkenness as a sin of the flesh that led to other fleshly sins, such as lust and gluttony. Again, Augustine emphasized the acute state of drunkenness as undesirable, especially as a result of consuming excessive wine in the context of Christian ritual. Apparently, he never made reference to drunkards, or chronically impaired drinkers.

Burton ([1621] 2000) provided some of the first indications that alcohol had a relationship with ongoing problems, and he asserted, somewhat incorrectly according to Abel (1999), that the ancients had identified "drunkards," or people given to excessive wine drinking. Informed by more accurate translation than that used by Burton, Abel indicates that, consistent with other information on the ancients' perceptions of wine and its consumption, the ancients' emphasis remained on the drunken episode rather than a chronic condition. The use of flawed translations may help explain why Keller (1979) so forcefully asserted in his overview of alcohol and alcoholism that the ancients understood alcoholism, but perhaps more influential in his interpretation of the ancients' writings about alcohol was his strong belief that alcoholism existed. Examples used by Keller to illustrate the ancients' concept of alcoholism (e.g., the fall from a rooftop of Odysseus's companion, Epenore, or a Greek eulogist's friend falling down) actually describe acute bouts of intoxication and their consequences, not chronic conditions of drunkenness.

Health and social ills associated with drinking alcoholic beverages appeared emphatically in William Hogarth's "Gin Lane" engraving released in 1751 (Rodin 1981:1238). The "gin mania" that swept the poor neighborhoods of London beginning about 1715 led to the development of patterned habitual drunkenness, abuse of families, and neglect and mistreatment of children. This response to high availability of gin was not lost on Hogarth, who sardonically depicted the alleged effects of that liquor on the poor people of London, including, it appears, facial deformities consistent with fetal alcohol syndrome. Even if the face of the poor baby being dropped to his death in that famous etching was only a product of Hogarth's outstanding observational acumen rather than any understanding of how the mother's drinking caused the baby's face to be misshapen, this point in Western history, one hundred years prior to Huss's introduction of the concept of alcoholism, marks the spot when alcohol use gained recognition in the West for its long-term consequences. If we also examine the social and economic conditions that produced Gin Lane, we find England making a transition to industrial capitalism with no constraints on the treatment of workers. Poor pay, squalid and overcrowded living conditions, and inter-class prejudice made the lives of people living in London's tenements sufficiently grim to warrant the consumption of very strong drink. A question raised by this development was how did the dominant sectors in society accept the increasingly inhuman conditions suffered by their fellow citizens? This question is fundamental to the purpose of this book as the Othering of the poor, expressed in the condemnation of their drug-using behaviors, served to justify their suffering as something they brought on themselves.

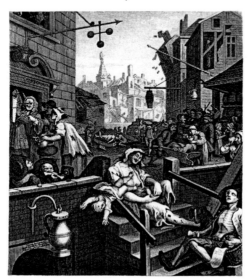

The beverage implicated in "gin lane" was qualitatively different from the wine and beer available to steady English drinkers before the introduction of distilled spirits by the Dutch in the seventeenth century (Fleming 1975). Whereas beer and wine provided the drinker with between four

Gin Lane (by William Hogarth, 1751)

and fourteen percent alcohol by volume, gin provided 40 percent, a truly efficient means of becoming intoxicated. Harkening back to the cytochrome P450 "shield" afforded by the herbivore forebears mentioned earlier, the availability of gin led to unprecedented stress on that system for processing alcohol in the liver. It is not surprising that astute observers such as Hogarth noticed poor health outcomes among the consumers of gin in his native England. He also contrasted gin lane with "beer street" in a second etching,

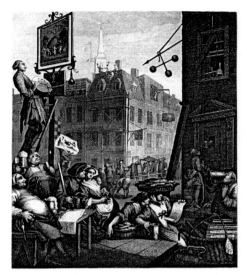

Beer Street (by William Hogarth, 1751)

showing prosperity, good health, and no endangered children in that illustration. In the relatively narrow span of 170 years, the bad reputation of distilled liquor, including blame for the dissolution of families, maltreatment of women and children, and ruination of personal finances had grown to the point where large numbers of people, particularly women, found the consumption of "hard" liquor intolerable and worthy of being eradicated. In fact, the time from when Magnus Huss gave a name to the condition of chronic drunk to the time when the United States ratified its 18th amendment prohibiting sale or production of alcoholic beverages only spanned 69 years, an astonishingly brief period in which a whole country (or at least two-thirds of the states) enacted prohibition of a widespread behavior. Given the rapidity with which it occurred after their introduction, one wonders if distilled spirits had not been invented and distributed whether prohibition would have happened at all.

OTHER DRUGS AND INTOXICATION

This question becomes a recurring theme as we examine the histories of other drugs in the human pharmacopoeia: Does the "refinement" of a drug's active ingredients always result in severe impact on the users? The beginnings of addiction as a concept appear to correspond in some cases to the refinement of certain basic drugs, including alcohol and tobacco, but the first important refinement of opioids, laudanum, pre-dates its acquiring a reputation for generating addicts by about three centuries. Paracelsus is credited with inventing this opium-based mixture in the early sixteenth century (Ball 2006), but use of opioid preparations in medicine can be traced to ancient Mesopotamia (Scarborough 2010:vii–4). The Greeks and Romans, including Hippocrates, Dioscorides, Nicander, Celsus, and Pliny all included opium in larger works that described various sectors of the ancient pharmacopoeia of their respective eras (Scarborough 2010:vii–5). Although the ancients apparently recognized the danger of poisoning from opium, and had fairly sophisticated methods for rendering it consumable, they did not report non-medical use of the drug. In England, as with distilled alcohol, public consciousness of laudanum as a problem lagged far behind its development as medicine. Thomas de Quincey's *Confessions of an English Opium Eater,* published in 1822, acknowledged that there were people in English society who had become habituated to a tincture of opium also called laudanum, but not the same as Paracelsus' formulation (Ball 2006:182-183), notably including some literati, as discussed in Chapter 4.

The production of the opium-alcohol tincture laudanum is credited to the British physician Thomas Sydenham (Davenport-Hines 2002:184). To make it, he prepared a concentration of the morphine alkaloid that was 25 times as potent as paregoric, achieving a potential for intoxication not possible through use of raw opium or other preparations available in the early 19th century. The fact that its invention did not engender a rapid rise in the number of impaired users is somewhat puzzling, considering the English response to gin and the uptake of cocaine in Europe within a couple of decades of the introduction of these concentrated drugs. Perhaps because laudanum's principal uses as anti-diarrhea and analgesic medicines, rather than pleasure-giving purposes, dominated medical applications, it simply did not occur to the recipients of laudanum in medical contexts to use the drug for anything other than alleviating symptoms. Concentrated alcohol in the form of rum or gin or brandy, on the other hand, went straight to the streets as a handy mitigation of stress and as a welcomed social lubricant. Despite its restricted medical pattern of use, potential addicts eventually "discovered" laudanum, although its heavy consumption never became as widespread as distilled ethyl alcohol.

THE "BIG FIVE" AND THEIR TRANSFORMATION INTO MORE DANGEROUS FORMS

The 19th century in Europe and the United States appears to have brought about a convergence of potent drug preparations which led ultimately to the development of the poly-drug configuration seen in present-day drug issues. In their concentrated forms, each presented new challenges to the metabolic capacities of their consumers, sometimes also producing patterns of highly recidivistic use. Five drugs in particular—alcohol, tobacco, opioids, cocaine, and cannabis became the principal components of Western drug consumption,[2] and all became, deservedly or not, associated with problems in the lives of their users. Each drug had a unique pathway toward widespread use and engendering problems among users. The following sections offer summaries of those pathways:

Alcohol. Distillation as a physical principle in the management of fluids was probably known to humans in the present-day Middle East as early as 1,100 years ago, but as noted earlier, its use in the production of preparations for general consumption did not become prevalent in Europe until sometime in the 17th century (Standage 2005: 94–95). Refinement of fermented liquids derived from sugar cane or grain became widespread as commerce with the West Indies and the rest of the world developed in Europe. Rum in particular became a currency in international trade with which slave traders plied their commerce in human misery and the British Empire compensated its sailors for services rendered and/or imposed. The New World bustled with activity in the invention, manufacture, distribution, and consumption of distilled beverages, including the sour mash concoctions of southern North America, rye whiskey in the north of that continent, and eventually, tequila in Mexico. The impact of their popularity, especially among males in the US populations, included the profusion of drinking houses, often called "saloons," and burgeoning social problems related to drunkenness that plagued the saloons' customers. The temperance movement in the United States was aimed at preventing the consequences of addiction to the powerful alcohol preparations sold in such establishments.

Tobacco. Nicotine is such a powerful drug that its dosage had to be reduced to make it a truly effective and heavily consumed commodity. The most widely used tobacco before the 19th century was in powdered form (snuff) as well as cut tobacco (which could be smoked in pipes, cigars, or hand-rolled cigarettes). Inhalation of pipe tobacco or cigars delivers such a jolt of nicotine that it induces nausea and dizziness. Hand rolling of small quantities of "mild" tobaccos into cigarettes required skill and patience that not many consumers had. In Spain in 1804, the introduction of hand-rolled "papeletes" constituted a first step in the eventual mass-production of ready-made tubes of cut tobacco from which smoke could be inhaled into the lungs, delivering a substantial dose of nicotine without dizzying toxic effects (Goodman 1993:90–99). These little vehicles of nicotine delivery could be carried around easily and consumed anywhere, and they were inexpensive enough to be used all the time. As the numbers of cigarette smokers grew and began in the 20th century to live long enough to incur cigarette-related illness, it became clear by 1964 that this product generated the most addictive tobacco consumption and the greatest hazard to the public health of any known drug.

Opioids. Opium, as we noted earlier, has been in the pharmacopoeia, beginning with people in the Fertile Crescent, for thousands of years, usually consumed as medicine for the treatment of pain, nausea, and diarrhea. It was a valuable medicine that could be used in very small quantities to treat patients for pain, coughing, or nausea. The introduction of water soluble preparations, including morphine sulfate and diacetyl morphine (heroin) in the 19th and 20th centuries eventually led to more widespread consumption of opioids (Musto 1987:1–3; Davenport-Hines 2002:184–187). Recently, nonmedical use of opioid analgesics of the next generation has emerged as a drug-use pattern of choice in many parts of the United States. Most prominent among these prescription preparations is Oxycontin, which is the brand name for a time-release version of the semi-synthetic preparation oxycodone, which in certain parts of the United States, has become popular and also dangerous, dominating emergency department statistics on accidental overdose.

Cannabis. Diffusion of this drug plant into the rest of the world traveled on two different historical tracks: (1) usage other than as a drug, and (2) use as a mind-altering drug. The former is apparently the more ancient, with some evidence of cannabis being used for food and fiber among the Chinese at least 3,500 years before the common era (BCE) (Booth 2003:17) The plant's long, pliant fibers constitute useful material for manufacturing cordage and clothing, and its fatty seeds are highly nutritious and totally devoid of the tetrahydrocannabinol that is the most pharmacologically active alkaloid in the plant. Almost as soon as the Spanish arrived in the New World, they attempted to encourage the planting of cannabis in most colonies (called Cáñamo). By the mid-sixteenth century, some cannabis plantations could be found as far south as Chile and as far north as Mexico (Carter et al. 1980:12). Nevertheless, in the New World, little evidence testifies to any form of cannabis use for mind-altering purposes until the 19th century. For psychotropic uses of cannabis, there was a different path, originating in India and traveling west into North Africa and Spain as the followers of Mohammed dominated the 8th through the 15th centuries in that part of the world. Reasons why it did not filter into Europe until the 19th century and never really became established in China are subject to conjecture, but alternative theories lack historical evidence. The European crusaders of the 11th through 13th centuries, despite the fact that many lived for extended periods in the "Holy Land" in the presence of hashish-smoking people, did not bring cannabis back to Europe with them. French soldiers under Napoleon, on the other hand, did. The wholesale shipping of indentured servants from India to Jamaica and Trinidad-Tobago provided another putative pathway for cannabis to enter the Western Hemisphere. Coming from an ancient tradition of cannabis use, the East Indians who were transferred to the West Indies likely brought their ganja with them, and, while they lived alongside African-descended populations, these immigrants imparted their patterns of drug consumption to their neighbors. All of the process described above is murky, because historians rarely attended to drug-using patterns of the poor and/or the populations of color. Nevertheless, by the beginning of the 20th century, the lands surrounding the Caribbean and the Gulf of Mexico were epicenters of diffusion of cannabis use into North America. Regarding potency of the preparations consumed, there was relatively little change between 800 and 1975, with a range of cannabis preparations' potency from bhang (drink made with bottom leaves of the plant) to ganja (tops and flowers of the female plant) to charas, or hashish (collected resin rich in THC). The latter form varied between 10 and 15 percent THC by weight. After 1975, as a broad market had been established, astute growers began to increase the THC content of cannabis through manipulation of hybrid strains and strategies to avoid formation of seeds (sinsemilla), edging the percentage of THC into content as high as 20 percent. It is uncertain whether this increase in potency has affected cannabis users in ways analogous to the apparent impact of distilled spirits, laudanum, and cocaine hydrochloride.

  Coca/cocaine. As early as 1800 BCE, natives of South America were cultivating coca. The plant had attracted their attention because someone had discovered that chewing its leaves gave feelings of well-being and satiation (Carter and Mamani 1986:69–70). That pattern of coca consumption spread throughout the Andes region, so that it was pervasive among mountain-dwelling people at the time of the Spanish conquest. The Spanish colonial administrators regarded coca chewing as a nasty habit of benighted indigenous people (Burchard 1976, 1992) but the behavior attracted the attention of European tourists who, upon noticing the strength, endurance, and energy of Aymara- and Quechua-speaking natives of the Andes in surroundings of high altitude, asked how they were able to function so well in the thin mountain air. The natives replied that coca enabled them to do these things. European chemists set about trying to discover what chemicals in the coca leaf might be pharmacologically active enough to cause the energy and strength they had observed. They were looking for the pharmacologically most active of the component compounds in the coca leaf, and they found one that was highly active and named it cocaine. In order to make this compound more readily useful as an ingredient in medicines, the chemists who isolated cocaine added a hydrochloride radical to make the alkaloid water soluble. Cocaine hydrochloride became a pervasive ingredient in the European and North American pharmacopoeias, primarily in energizing elixirs. It also became useful as a local anesthetic for facial surgery. Before long, large numbers of North American housewives were addicted to the elixirs. Freud had briefly endorsed the drug as a treatment for depression and later recanted. The short half-life of its acute effects and the spiraling patterns that its use engenders have caused various cocaine epidemics to wax and wane over the century-and-a-half that this drug has been available. Between 2009 and 2011 it again was object of a surge in popularity in both Europe and the United States among youth who came of age in the 21st Century.

In addition to the Big Five drugs mentioned above, methamphetamine emerged as a drug of choice in certain parts of the United States by the beginning of the 21st Century. It has a much shorter history than any of the big five, being isolated in 1893 and scheduled in 1944 as a pharmaceutical drug in the United States, specific for narcolepsy and exogenous obesity. Methamphetamine use as a recreational drug became pervasive in parts of the North American Midwest, West, and Southeast by the year 2000. In 2008, methamphetamine was about 6 percent of the drugs mentioned in emergency-department presentations that involved drugs (DAWN 2009). This figure places methamphetamine ahead of all other drugs in the second tier of drugs (those not part of the Big Five). Its potential for engendering addiction gained recognition during the 1960s, if not earlier. Along with its close relative, amphetamine, methamphetamine developed a following of devotees who earned a separate designation: "speed freaks" which gained common usage by the late 1960s. The people known to use these highly active stimulants acquired a reputation for obsessive, repetitive use of their drugs of choice, by any ingestion route possible, although the injection route appeared to be especially favored. The gloss that denoted this kind of drug user carried clear implications of ongoing use and extreme disruption of normal behavior patterns.

We cannot achieve the same precision in defining exactly when the drugs included in the Big Five (or Six) became associated specifically with a separate kind of human being involved in the obsessive pursuit of that particular drug. That, however, is exactly the kind of question that this chapter, and more broadly, this book seeks to answer. How and when did some human beings come to define a set of human beings as Others based on their long-term, regular consumption of a specific drug? In the preceding discussion, the evidence suggests that a concept of "addict" or "(fill in the addictive drug or activity)-holic" is not very old in the total history of humankind, perhaps as little as 200-years old, a phenomenon we here label *social externalization*. It is based on the identification of people within a social body who are defined on the basis of their use of drugs (or participation in other disapproved activities) as inherently different and as threatening and their subjection to rituals of social rejection and attacks on their social worth. In the case of drug-related addiction, the concept appears to be related to the refinement of drug preparations into highly concentrated forms capable of engendering craving and compulsive use. All of these developments seem to converge during the 19th century, so that, by 1900, it was possible to be recognized by your fellow human beings as an alcoholic or a person addicted to morphine and/or cocaine. At that time, tobacco cigarettes were gaining popularity and were on the verge of being mass manufactured by machines and promoted by governments and what were soon to be very wealthy national and trans-national corporations (Singer 2008). Although some evidence indicates that people in North America and Western Europe began to recognize the addictive potential of tobacco long before the introduction of ready-made cigarettes (Goodman 1993), cigarettes became the most convenient method for ingesting nicotine and ultimately, the most deadly.

The most-refined forms of cannabis, charas and hashish, were already ancient by 1800, but were not well known outside of India and the Middle East. Cannabis did, however, migrate to Europe and the New World in the 19th century, eventually diffusing in a limited way from migration focal points in France and Jamaica, respectively. Those who took up cannabis use in France included the veterans of Napoleon's invasion of Egypt and eventually members of the literati, such as Dumas and Baudelaire (1971:70–71). In the case of Indian ganja and its migration to the Caribbean there is no evidence of any preparations other than teas, infusions (that were not mind altering but medicinal), and smokable plant material in any of the 19th century accounts of cannabis use in the New World. Ethnographic accounts of ganja use in Jamaica (cf. Dreher 1982; Rubin and Comitas 1975) report no forms of cannabis use other than either boiling or smoking the plant's leaves, tops, and flowers. Some evidence of a recent trend may appear in the statistics on drug-treatment presentations, in which cannabis is a leading drug of choice in the self-reports of new treatment patients (Schensul et al. 2000). Skepticism may be appropriate in interpreting these figures, however, because of the young (14–17) age of the presenting patients and the fact that they often are referred to treatment by their parents or their schools.

Regardless of the degree to which people who present for treatment of problems related to cannabis use can be assessed as addicts, it is clear that this particular drug did not develop as strong a reputation for causing drug-related problems as did alcohol, opioids, and cocaine during a key period of Western history between 1700 and 1900. In fact, cannabis was essentially absent from discussions of drug-induced impairment as the reputations for addictive problems of the other three were growing most rapidly. In Western Europe, Baudelaire's coterie hardly elicited a response other than bemusement at the outlandish reports of intoxicated experiences that they produced. Emerging news of "soldiers' disease," afflicting thousands of veterans who sustained war wounds in 19th-century wars, the widely read "confessions" by DeQuincey describing the life trajectory of an addict, and reports of cocaine-addicted housewives in the United States attracted much more public attention than a handful of French bohemians' dabbling in cannabis use. In fact, there has developed a certain degree of social expectation that artists and intellectuals will engage in borderline behaviors without suffering the full weight of opprobrium to which others are subjected, especially if they come from subordinated social classes. To a degree, it appears, they are allowed to walk on the wild side as a means of providing vicarious pleasure to the constrained masses.

Human susceptibility to habituation or addiction remains something of an enigma, yet it is highly relevant to the question of how people come to be perceived as addicts. Why are people affected so variously by the consumption of the drugs? Most people who ever use alcohol or opioids or cocaine do not become alcoholics or addicts, but some do. What sets those who do apart from those who do not? Ming Tsuang and colleagues (1998) attempted to investigate this question from the point of view afforded by the sector of behavioral genetics known as twin studies. Using data collected from 7,500 male twin pairs, this investigative team set out to determine how much of the potential to have problems with drugs involved heredity. Not surprisingly, they found that they could explain about half of the variance in the presence or absence of drug-related problems in terms of genetic background and half in terms of environment. This result was not surprising because studies going back to Vaillant (1983) have found more or less the same thing. For the present discussion, however, the more interesting part of Tsuang et al.'s findings is that the genetic component characterized by their studies was generic in terms of the addict's or problem user's drug of choice. In other words, people with exactly the same genetic makeup (i.e., monozygotic, or "identical" twins) could develop problematic use of any or all of the Big Five drugs in any configuration (e.g., cigarettes, alcohol, and cocaine, or marihuana, tobacco, and heroin). Social environment was found to influence specific drug choices, but genetic makeup helped determine whether or not the individual would have problems with his drugs of choice (Tsuang et al. 1998). In this sense, then, the addict or problematic drug user is in fact qualitatively unlike his/her contemporaries in terms of genetic makeup, which in part causes him/her to respond to psychotropic drugs differently, namely more intensely. If certain drug preparations were modified to deliver their key mind-altering ingredients (e.g., ethanol, morphine, or cocaine) in more concentrated form than they had ever done in the history of their use by humans, that concentration in combination with a genetic predisposition to feel that concentration intensely would be likely to produce a reaction beyond what had been possible previously. Tsuang et al. suggest that a subset of humans have the predisposition to feel drugs—any of the Big Five—more forcefully than the rest of us. The introduction of highly potent forms of the Big Five would have a high likelihood of matching drug consumption with this kind of predisposition.

Again, the biological part of the analysis only explains half of the variance (and, it should be noted, none of the social reaction to heavy drug use). Environmental factors explain the other half. Exposure to cultural contexts in which potent drugs are used is a crucial variable in the establishment of addictive patterns, especially if the use pattern itself is highly frequent and heavy. Clearly, inner-city London was such an environment by 1750. Harlem in the 1960s was also, as was East Harlem of the 1980s. In each of these places—and socially defined place is hence an important issue—people internalized a vague cultural idea that they were equal with everyone else in society, but yet their daily experiences in interaction with other people told them that they were in fact unequal and did not count. They received poor wages for hard work and had few prospects of transcending their social place because of clogged opportunity structures. In these conditions of social derogation, resorting to strong drink or potent drugs could be seen as a strategy to get through inevitably unpleasant days and self-recriminating nights. Adoption of heavy, chronic patterns of consuming cheap, abundant drugs became widespread, and the proliferation of heavy users invited generalizations about the nature of the drug-using population at large. Given the recently achieved potency of the drugs of choice, by the late 1800s, the stage was set for the identification of addicts, especially poor addicts, but to a certain extent all addicts as separate subpar categories of human being.

NOTES

1 Nothing of that antiquity has been found so far in the New World—probably because there were no fruits quite as sugar-laden as *Vitis vinifera sylvestris*. Corn and Agave were early contributors to the production of fermented beverages, but the evidence of their domestication is much later (ca. 1500 BCE, compared with 5000–6000 BCE for the Old World). The evidence also depends on residues in stone or clay containers, which appear later in the New World than the Old. In all likelihood humans discovered plant-derived preparations of some kind much earlier than the evidence for corn and agave would testify, but the accoutrements of these preparations left no trace from which to infer use.

2 Because they are 20th century drugs without the same historical background of being associated with problems of chronic use and addiction, we have not included LSD or methamphetamine in this group. By the time those drugs were synthesized and introduced into consumption, the concept of addiction was already well established. Otherwise, methamphetamine certainly would be a candidate for inclusion, based on its accelerating reputation as an addictive drug. LSD, on the other hand, is not really associated with addiction at all.

CHAPTER THREE

Representations of Addicts and the Construction of Prohibitions

T
o what extent did public awareness of drug consumption's negative impact on drug users and their families and others around them lead to the formation of public opinion against alcohol and other drugs? Was alcoholism as prevalent in the streets of London as Hogarth would have had us believe? What did the advocates of temperance find so abhorrent about the behavior of drunks that they wanted to abolish all alcoholic beverages? Why did they think they could do so in light of cultural values about personal freedom? All of these questions reflect the struggle with how powerful attitudes of intolerance come to dominate in societies that accept in their midst many different ways of life and systems of belief. This chapter focuses on the temperance movements in the United Kingdom and the United States, primarily because the history of those movements is so thoroughly documented, but partly because both polities were in the process of either managing or establishing world-encircling empires. In fact, the impetus for extending moral and religious influence to an international level appears to have driven the American Temperance movement and influenced the international conventions banning "dangerous" drugs (Tyrrell 1991; 2010). The discussion begins by attempting to explain how people come to the point of consigning other people to a separate and lower category than themselves, based on an often highly skewed reading of the others' behavior patterns. We assert that this process involves attribution, in which people count themselves as distinct from other people based on complexes of behavior observed in the Others that they find, as a result of the cultural meanings they carry, to be abhorrent or worthy of derogation. For example, at a time of growing fears about terrorism, Sikhs in the United States, a group that previously may have been perceived as exotic but harmless, suddenly were subject to increasing incidence of violent attacks as they were assigned to the general cultural category of dangerous, head-gear wearing, foreign Others. Sociological theories, such as "labeling" and "strain" add a layer of social process to this kind of thinking about others. Two historically important places where

The Social Value of Drug Addicts: The Uses of the Useless, by Merrill Singer and J. Bryan Page, 71–87.

people engaged in this kind of thinking about Others were England and the United States, as they had the power to spread their ideas globally. This chapter traces the inchoate processes of Othering as they occurred in these nations, starting with temperance movements in the early 19th century, and culminating in the establishment of public houses in Great Britain and the experiment with prohibition in the United States.

THE ORIGINS OF OTHERING

The process of vilifying not just a behavior but a category of persons who engage in a specific pattern of consuming drugs had its beginnings in the public discourse on the ills associated with consumption of alcoholic beverage, especially in contexts of material deprivation and moral disorientation. One key to this process was, and still is, attribution. People who considered themselves to be "normal" began to view the lifestyles, behaviors, and values of a set of people in plain sight as both unacceptable and not normal. In so doing, they attributed intemperance, impulsivity, hedonism, and normlessness to people living in circumstances of poverty whose primary strategy for coping with hopelessness involved strong drink. Another key to this process of derogating other people is separation. It is easy to attribute undesirable characteristics to people whose way of life is largely unknown and but presumably different from that of the attributor. In fact, the combination of separation and attribution attracted the attention of sociologists, who built theories about this process of separation and attribution, variously called "deviance" (Becker 1963), "labeling" (Becker 1963), "strain"(Cloward and Ohlin 1960), and "differential association" (Cressey 1962) among others (Cohen 1955). One of the logical dilemmas in these theories involves the question of precedence—what preceded what? Did some kind of collectively recognized experience occur in which the surrounding un-labeled groups recognized patterns of undesirable behavior among those being labeled? Did the labeling groups simply decide, based on differences between them and the groups being labeled, to bestow the label on a group they did not like?

If we look back into the beginnings of separation and attribution as they took place during the 18th century in England, we can recognize strong opinions formed by physicians regarding the nature of alcohol consumption as a kind of sickness. Benjamin Rush, a signatory of the Declaration of Independence, was one of the American physicians who articulated a perception that the habitual drunkard could not help him/herself when confronted with the possibility of consuming alcohol (Levine 1978). Rush, however, was not the only physician to take this view of spirituous liquors and their effects on humankind. Levine (1978) wrote that the early temperance movement could rightly be called a physicians' temperance movement because of the involvement of physicians who had seen first-hand the effects of repeated drunkenness. Rush led the movement, published his clinical findings, and asserted that anyone could be victimized by the consumption of liquor. He also declared that the only remedy for this affliction was total abstinence. Not-so-coincidentally, similar views on opioids developed in England at the same time. Rush began publishing his temperance pamphlets at the turn of the 19th Century, and de Quincey published his *Confessions of an English Opium Eater* in 1822.

This timing, in light of the evidence presented in the previous chapter, has significance as a sign of a shift in public discourse in the West on intoxicants and the people who consume them frequently. No longer were drunken behaviors momentary events in the lives of otherwise "normal" people. They carried new meaning and portent as the unintoxicated tried to discern whether or not an episode of intoxication signified a chronic problem—akin to a disease. The socioeconomic circumstances of becoming drunk or high also received scrutiny, leading to the generation of causal theories constructed to explain the occurrence of abject poverty, abuse of children and spouses, and ultimately disease and death. These theories were not purely the products of inductive accumulation of facts about the dangers of addiction by physicians. They gathered powerful impetus from their proponents' attitudes about class, character, and moral behavior (Seddon 2010:62; Tyrrell 2010:21). Furthermore, Tyrrell holds that the temperance movement was just one of several larger issues involving the United States' expansive desire to "reform the world" in many different aspects of the human condition. The issues promoted by North American world campaigners included adhering to Christianity, banning prostitution, giving up nonwestern or working-class lifestyles, improving hygiene, and generally achieving moral purity (Tyrrell 2010:21). This desire to achieve absolute reform will receive further attention later in this chapter. The word "temperance" deserves some discussion here, as it became the standard label for all organizations and persons who wished to limit or curtail alcohol consumption in their respective societies, both in England and in the United States. In the case of England, the temperance groups' original agenda was to convince people not to drink to the point of drunkenness—in other words—to drink in a temperate fashion. Some participants in the movement, perhaps recognizing that established heavy drinkers had great difficulty stopping, and were likely to suffer recidivism if they took a drink after becoming sober, began to demand that alcohol be banned completely from English society. "Temperance," then, had in their eyes become undesirable, because it placed at risk former drinkers. In the end, as we shall see, temperance won out in England. Amid the generalized reformist zeal in the United States, the word "temperance" remained an important label of the anti-alcohol movement, despite the fact that practically all of the movement's adherents would settle for nothing less than a constitutional amendment enacting total prohibition of alcohol and hence they were really prohibitionists.

THE TEMPERANCE MOVEMENT IN ENGLAND

This movement emerged in the late 18th century, and by the 1830s, it had momentum. The following historic tract, made available online, gives the reader a sense of the tone employed by 19th century campaigners in England against the vices that would later be called addictions:

> The habitual opium eater is instantly recognized [sic] by his appearance. A total attenuation of body, and a withered yellow countenance, a lame gait, and a bending of the spine, frequently to such a degree as to assume a circular form, and glossy, deep, sunken eyes betray him at first glance. The digestive organs are in the highest degree disturbed, the sufferer eats scarcely anything, and has hardly had an evacuation in a week; his mental and physical powers are destroyed—he is impotent (Anonymous 1845?).

This writer describes stereotypically the condition of the thoroughly impaired opium eater, emphasizing the physical deterioration thought to ensue inevitably after forming the habit of consuming laudanum. The same source took a dim view of tobacco as well as inserting racist commentary about the production of cigars:

> If the processes by which cigars are rolled together by the filthy and sweaty hands of negroes in Havannah [sic] aided by occasional applications of saliva to make the leaves adhere, were more generally known, it would excite as much disgust against smoking as against chewing; and both of these habits, as well as that of stuffing the nostrils with tobacco powder are so truly dirty ... (Anonymous 1845?).

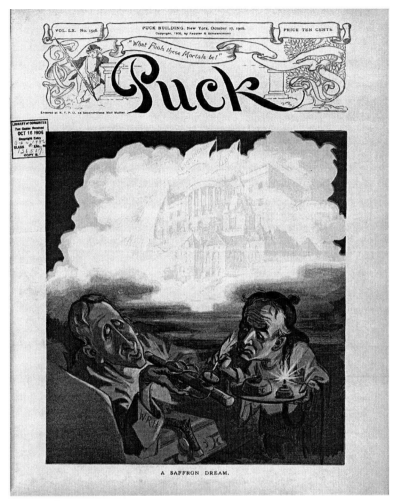

Opium dream

Whoever wrote the tract containing these excerpts completely disapproved of the people who engaged in this behavior that he/she intended to stamp out. Consumption of alcohol, however, was the real target of the tract, and in the section addressing alcohol, the attribution of social ills becomes truly extravagant.

> A large proportion of pauperism, loss of health and character; premature death, widowhood and orphanage; abandonment to vicious

pursuits and crimes; an enormous outlay in supporting judicial tribu-
nals, police establishments, jails, and penal settlements; the abstraction
of land from useful crops for food; and the distraction of capital into
wrong channels. Of the evils ensuing under the head of public morals
and religion, the picture is too appalling to be dwelt upon (Anonymous
1845?).

By the time that this tract likely was written, animus had accumulated
against the perceived evils of all the accused drugs for at least 50 years, and
the tract's author's vehemence reflects that animus. The final sentence, after
having enumerated serious problems attributed to alcohol, says that the loss
of health, leaving of widows and orphans, criminality, and waste of resources
the writer just mentioned is not nearly as horrifying as the alcohol-caused
moral degradation he/she refuses to describe. Elsewhere in the same tract,
the author declares the goal of eliminating tobacco, opioids, and alcohol from
English society. This attitude emanates from the notion that no human being
can avoid becoming habituated to these and other drug preparations if they
have so much as a single taste of them. Therefore, according to this view, the
drug preparations mentioned in the tract and any others that might intoxicate
humans must be eliminated completely from human society. This teetotal
approach to what would eventually be called prohibition would brook no
space for moderate uses of tobacco, alcohol, and opioids.

Another, somewhat briefer tract written by the Reverend William Wight
(Wight 1845?) cites a succinct (if confused) expression of the same notion:
"The temperate are the chief promoters of drunkenness" (Wight 1845?: 4).
Did not the Scottish Temperance League identify "temperance" as a desirable
goal? "The temperate," however, are blamed for drunkenness. The phrase
meant to express displeasure at those who maintained that alcohol could be
consumed moderately, i.e. temperately. Wight's own choice of words favors
another term, as in his tract, the word "drunkard" appears many times, and
its usage carries the implication of "lost soul." Wight proceeds to assert that
the vast majority of Scottish society consists of drunkards. He also attributes
the apparent closing of Welsh churches to the drinking proclivities of their
pastors. Wight also indicts the working class for intemperance in consumption of strong drink, citing Birmingham and Glasgow:

Take Birmingham, the workshop of England; notwithstanding all
the clamours of the people about taxation and depression of trade,
it appears the people of that town are spending £600,000 annually

in strong drink. At Glasgow, a committee was appointed some time back to inquire into the causes of distress so prevalent; and it came out in evidence that £1,200,000 were annually spent in that city in intoxicating liquors, of which sum the working-classes spent *one million* (Wight 1845?: 6).

That the English working class had essentially self-inflicted their miserable state in 19th century became a prevailing attitude among those who expressed concern about the pauperization of families associated with recidivistic heavy drinking. Of course, neither the good Reverend Wight nor his Temperance Society colleagues had conducted the studies necessary to establish strong drink as a cause of poverty (or vice-versa, for that matter). In fairness to them, the expertise necessary to conduct rigorous studies of this kind was at least 80 years in the future, but commentators like Wight could cite years of inductive observations to buttress their views. Nevertheless, the onus of what could be called a pandemic of drinking problems in mid-19th century England was placed fully on the shoulders of the working class, leaving them to take additional blame for the deplorable conditions in which they lived.

Who were the people who accused the urban poor of profligate spending on alcohol, inattention to hygiene and home, and moral decay? It is relatively easy to recall the Woman's Christian Temperance Union as a movement that exerted influence on the eventual ratification in the United States of Amendment 18, prohibiting production, sale, and consumption of alcoholic beverages in the United States, but who were these people in England? Were they housewives? Full-time moral crusaders? Upper-class social leaders? Friedrich Engels certainly was not one of them, as his works in 1846 and 1872 took the approach of examining structural factors, such as the process of enclosure, the crowding of impoverished workers in urban tenements, and the oppressive conditions in which the poor earned inadequate wages (Engels 1845[2001]). Nevertheless, his voice against class-based structural violence as the likely cause of London's terrible inner city conditions and rampant gin consumption had little influence in England's political landscape (Singer 1986).

Joseph Livesey (1794–1884) was one of the British temperance movement's most steadfast proponents in the 19th century. He co-organized the movement's first meetings at the time of its inception in 1832 (Carter 1933). Orphaned at age seven and sent to live with his grandfather, Livesey learned how to work in his grandfather's tiny (three looms) basement textile mill at an early age. As he matured, he developed his own business producing cheese.

Throughout his life, he spoke up against misery and injustice wherever he saw it, and in northern England in the early 19th century he had plenty of things to speak against—enclosure, poor wages, crowded housing, and debtors' prison, to name a few. In the process of growing up and continuing to live among the poor people of London, he came to perceive spirituous liquors as a curse of humankind.

Two years before the first temperance movement meeting, in response to growing sentiment that beer was being too heavily controlled and taxed, Parliament passed the Beerhouse Act in an effort to encourage more cultivation of barley and hops and more manufacture of beer. The act's framers had been concerned about the ongoing epidemic of gin consumption and felt that greater availability of beer might reduce consumption of gin (Carter 1933:25). According to Carter's (1933) account, they were disastrously mistaken. Beer houses proliferated in response to this Act, and, believing themselves to be in competition with the beer houses, the gin-serving establishments stepped up their promotions and advertising, sometimes upgrading facilities to attract their clientele. The impact on the street of these developments was the widespread appearance of public drunkenness. The following narrative paints a picture of how badly the Act proceeded in the case of an establishment that had been recently renovated in response to the Act's provisions:

> A band of music was stationed in front of the house; the street became almost impassable from the number of people collected; and when the doors were opened, the rush was tremendous; it was instantly filled with customers, and continued so till midnight.... We found that all the other gin palaces were equally crowded as before; they had all lowered their prices to compete with this new shop, and attracted a large number of customers (Carter 1933:29).

Indeed, the primary impact of the Beerhouse Act appears to have been to make alcoholic beverages more accessible than before the Act.

Harkening back to Hogarth's etchings, one might ask, why so much public drunkenness, if much of the consumption was beer? Wasn't beer supposedly the drink of gentle intoxication, not leading to ruinous drunkenness? The answer may lie in the impact of gin as the beverage that intoxicated people in a way they had not been intoxicated before. Gin and rum were the first spirituous liquors of high potency to be widely available and cheap, allowing a large proportion of the population the opportunity to experience being drunk. Furnas (1965: 65–66) asserted that people could get drunk on fermented drinks ever since the New Stone Age, and thus the blame placed by early temperance advocates on hard liquor was misdirected. According to Furnas (1965), the idea of teetotal prohibition emanated from the realization that any and all alcoholic beverages could produce drunkenness. In fact, as Chapter 2 explains, people did not apply a concept of chronicity to drunkenness until sometime after 1500, as spirituous liquors became available (Gusfield 1996:91). Gin and rum made it very easy to get drunk, and once people had become drunk and decided they liked the experience, they continued to pursue drunkenness by whatever means was available to them.

If beer were more available than gin or rum, that availability could lead part of the heavy drinkers' market toward getting drunk on beer. The wide availability of really cheap and convenient beer may help to explain the Beerhouse Act's outcome. Gin represented a pathway for discovering and practicing drunkenness, but once discovered and practiced, any source of alcohol would do in pursuit of its reoccurrence. This process was actually a question of probability. People drinking distilled spirits were significantly more likely than people drinking beer or wine to drink well past the point of the two-drink "buzz," also known as the "potentiating dose." If the ones who drank enough gin or rum to become drunk found that experience to be gratifying they could be expected to try to repeat it with whatever alcoholic preparation was at hand.

The sequence of events after the passage of the Beerhouse Act had the net effect of galvanizing the resolve of temperance advocates whose primary agenda was moral reform of British society. According to activists like Livesey, the mere presence of alcoholic beverage in the community was sufficient to bring about widespread drunkenness and ruinous behavior. He and his followers held that total abstinence represented the only way to avoid the ill effects of alcoholic beverages, and they formulated pledges that articulated the fundamental principle of avoiding all forms of alcohol:

> I do voluntarily promise that I will abstain from ale, porter, wine cider, ardent spirits, or any other intoxicating liquors, and that I will not give nor offer them to others, except as medicine or in a religious ordinance; and that I will discountenance all the cause and practices of intemperance (Carter 1933:253).

On the resolve of abstainers who took the pledge cited above and considerable support from the United States' temperance movement, the World's Temperance Convention took place in England in 1846, with hopes of galvanizing world opinion in favor of banning alcoholic beverages (Tyrrell 2010). The British side of the temperance movement, however, aimed for somewhat more moderate goals than their North American counterparts. They never succeeded in moving the English government toward full banning of alcoholic beverages, but they nevertheless succeeded, through the Wine and Beerhouse Act of 1869, in instituting the licensing of public houses whose hours of business were regulated and whose licensing was a matter for national governance. The English prohibitionists conducted a series of legislative skirmishes in their attempts to enact a local option veto, so that individual communities could ban public houses from their premises (Carter 1933: 199), since a national ban was not in the offing. This activity never succeeded, and consequently, the ancient and venerable English tradition of going to the "local" to raise a pint with one's mates continued uninterrupted. In 2005, the serving laws limiting hours and distribution of licenses were liberalized.

PROHIBITION IN THE UNITED STATES

In the United States, on the other hand, abstentionists achieved success beyond Livesey's wildest dreams. Their travails have received attention in Ken Burns's television chronicle, *Prohibition,* as well as Szymanski's *Pathways to Prohibition* (2003) and Tyrrell's *Reforming the World* (2010) among many other works. Here, we explore the motivations, tactics, and outcomes of the prohibitionists to try to understand how they accomplished the massive, daunting and unlikely task of getting two-thirds of the states to ratify a complete ban on alcoholic beverages.

The local option veto also was tried by the American prohibitionists in various forms at various levels of government. Much of this activity took place in the 1890s, and by the time of the final push toward ratification of the 18th amendment, it had become clear that local option vetoes were not going to succeed. Prohibitionists eventually concluded that an amendment to the Federal constitution would be preferable (Szymanski 2003:91). Besides, the local ordinances would have resulted in a patchwork that could be easily evaded by using differences in neighboring jurisdictions' ordinances for purposes of trafficking in and serving alcoholic drinks (a pattern that continues to exist in various parts of the United States with local alcohol control ordinances).

But why this zeal for keeping all alcoholic beverages away from all people in the United States? What was it about alcohol that had the prohibitionists so exercised? It seems that the perceived impact of drunkenness on social order and the sanctity of the family had strong influence on public opinion. The overall rate at which early Euro-Americans consumed liquor has been estimated at some seven gallons per year per person in the years between 1790 and 1840 (Salinger 2002: 2). Current figures fall somewhat short of that amount, although comparison requires a bit of conversion into liters of absolute (100 percent) alcohol. If we estimate that those seven gallons were 40 percent alcohol by volume, and using figures of 128 ounces per gallon and 33.8 ounces per liter, that amounts to 10.6 liters per person per year. Estimates provided by the World Health Organization place US consumption of alcohol at 8.5 liters per person per year (WHO 2004: 12). Despite the strong likelihood that a higher proportion of the U.S population drinks now than did at the turn of the 19th century, and given the increase in women drinkers, individual North American drinkers drink less overall than they did two centuries ago. Because men predominated among drinkers in the late 18th and early 19th centuries, those who drank were probably taking in prodigious quantities of alcohol. Given the available descriptions of that era's alcohol consumption patterns (see Furnas 1965), there is no reason to doubt that some men spent at least part of every day drunk.

The so-called "culture wars" often invoked in present-day discourse to denote clashes in world view within North American society are nothing new. Gusfield (1996:10) points out that similar clashes occurred in the United States during the latter half of the 19th century, pitting segments of a predominantly white non-Hispanic population against each other on the basis of Protestant, rural world view versus Catholic- and Jew-inclusive, urban world view. In the process of marshaling forces for this clash, problems related to alcohol use were framed as an issue that required total intolerance of alcoholic beverages in order to improve social conditions. This approach to pathologizing all alcohol use dismissively discounted the ways in which Italian Catholics, Irish Catholics, and Jews drank beer and wine in contexts where those drinks were considered part of food and its consumption, and in many cases, also part of sacred ritual. Alcohol consumption, in the vast majority of instances, then and now, does not lead to the kind of chronic intoxication that afflicts alcohol addicts, yet the prohibitionists, as described earlier, conceived of any alcohol use as inevitably leading down a slippery slope to eventual impairment, ill health, financial ruin, immorality, and child neglect.

Unfortunately for the forces opposing prohibition, two factors worked against them: (1) the pervasiveness of grim case histories describing the human damage associated with heavy alcohol consumption and (2) the ability of print media to present these case histories to a reading public that was far more extensive than ever before. Practically every adult living in 19th century England or the United States had, in his/her repertoire of stories, at least one about a man who, in a state of intoxication, had committed some heinous act of violence or reckless endangerment. By the mid-19th century, these stories no longer remained localized, but if they were particularly poignant or entertaining, could disseminate across the nation by means of print media (Behr 2011: 63–64).

Benjamin Rush (1786), in his *Enquiries* writings, was early to weigh in on the ruinous effects of hard liquor on families:

> Spirits impair the memory, debilitate the understanding, and pervert the moral faculties ... [and they] produce not only falsehood, but fraud, theft, uncleanliness, and murder. ... How deep the anguish which rends the bosom of the [drunkard's] wife ... the shame and aversion which she excites in her husband! Is he the father of children? See their averted looks ... their blushing looks at each other! (Rush 1786).

This printed tract tapped into its readership's personal experience, because the readers had seen similar phenomena in their immediate social environments. It was also designed, as are the altar calls in some church services, to draw the person whose own family life has resembled the one described into the realization that they need to stop drinking. This example, however, is relatively mild, and reflects an almost clinical perspective on the effect of heavy drinking on the drinker's family. According to Furnas (1965) the next fifty years saw the emergence of far more powerful and enflamed narratives than this, delivered by talented and manipulative orators such as John B. Gough, the Reverend Theobald Mathew, General Neal Dow, and the first Prohibition Party candidate for president of the United States, General John P. St. John (Furnas 1965:128–129). Their strident tone escalated throughout the 19th century, exhorting their audiences to "take the pledge" and encourage their peers to do so.

The mid-19th century in the United States was a time of contested ways of life, not just with regard to the question of prohibiting alcohol, but also on the question of slavery. Furnas (1965) features a parallelism between the most widely read prohibitionist writer, Timothy Shay Arthur, and the famous abolitionist, Harriett Beecher Stowe. In Furnas's analysis, the two activists shared a "watery" quality in their writing, but at the same time a certain power to manipulate the feelings of their readers. Arthur's portfolio was at least as extensive as Stowe's, which included 22 books, of which *Uncle*

Tom's Cabin was the most widely read . Arthur's books were very diverse, including writings on housekeeping, mothering, retirement, career building, paths to prosperity, and marriage (Furnas 1965:126). His most influential book, however, focused on the evils of alcohol. Arthur's *Ten Nights in a Bar-Room* gave readers an elaborate narrative on how the presence of a tavern in a community sets in motion terrible processes, including murder, injury of children, deterioration of a business, fall of a public official, and the inevitable delirium tremens (DTs). In all likelihood, Arthur was far more familiar with the setting of his novel than Stowe, who lived in Connecticut, was with the location of *Uncle Tom's Cabin.* Arthur's descriptions of activities and operations of the Sickle and Sheaf, the fictitious bar in which his story is set, bespeak familiarity with bars and their clientele (Furnas 1965:129). After the Civil War, Arthur wrote several other novels of equally propagandist intent: *The Bar-Rooms at Brantly, Three Years in a Man-Trap, The Strike at Tivoli Mills,* and *Danger* (Furnas 1965:128). Decades after the release of *Ten Nights,* with prohibitionist activity at a fever pitch in 1890, the book's copyright expired, making possible the distribution of thousands of copies by prohibitionist activists at 25 cents each.

During the 19th century's period of escalating rhetoric against alcoholic beverages, the concept of delirium tremens became a popular tool for convincing prohibitionist audiences of the ills that drinking visits upon drinkers (Furnas 1965 119–120). Every prohibitionist or temperance lecturer had his/her standard story of the pink elephants, little green men, and snakes of assorted colors seen by drunks who had withdrawn (or had been withdrawn) from alcohol. The lecturers vividly described the tortured souls who had screamed all night, terrified of the hallucinations, cold sweats, nausea, and convulsions, and who begged for relief of any kind from their torment. There was much truth to these accounts, as withdrawal from alcohol by a true alcohol addict is perhaps the most torturous and life-threatening of all withdrawal syndromes. Nevertheless, the presentations by prohibitionists usually failed to report that, in order to reach the point in a drinking career where withdrawal symptoms occur, it is necessary for an adult to be drinking in excess (i.e., over five drinks a day) for an extended period of time and then stop or drastically reduce alcohol consumption (Erwin et al. 1998; Rosenbaum et al. 1940). A history of drinking heavily and experiencing other kinds of alcohol withdrawal symptoms may eventually lead to delirium tremens in up to 5 percent of patients who withdraw from alcohol use abruptly. This condition is sometimes fatal, with a death rate that has yet to improve over the 5–15 percent rate originally noted in the early 1800s, despite efforts to develop better treatment techniques (Erwin et al.1998). The prohibitionists' discourse during the 19th century, however, implied that any and all drinkers would be subject to DTs in short order and without exception. Furnas (1965:120) provides an example of this kind of discourse when he quotes the well-meaning Dr. Hale:

> Temperance got good service from DTs, even maintaining that this fulminating neuropsychiatric disaster is not confined to heavy drinkers "[Y]ou are not as safe as you imagine," the American Temperance Society told the occasional imbiber. " Some of the worst cases of (DTs) ... have been of persons who had rarely or never been known to be intoxicated ... and were regarded by their neighbors as temperate men." ... Temperance could always find well-meaning doctors eager to lie in the good cause (Furnas 1965:120).

The forces for prohibition used vilification of the sellers of alcoholic beverages as another rhetorical tactic as the campaign against strong drink heated up. This development seemed inevitable as women swelled the ranks of the prohibitionist faithful. During the 19th century in North America, saloons had almost exclusively male clientele. Consequently, they tended to be viewed by women as places where men were up to no good, a perception that was hardly unwarranted, given the numbers of women who had the experience of receiving men home from the saloon broke, belligerent, impotent, and unmanageable. Therefore, the prohibitionists reasoned, the person who owns and runs such establishments must be intentionally evil. In a quote from John Wesley, the saloon keepers were "poisoners general ... [including] all who sell liquor in the common way.... They murder his Majesty's subjects by wholesale ... drive them to hell like sheep" (Furnas 1965:122). Lyman Beecher, another outspoken prohibitionist, also aimed a blanket accusation of murder at all saloon owners. He defied "any man who understands the nature of ardent spirit, and yet for the sake of gain, continues to be engaged in the traffic, to show that he is not involved in the crime of murder" (Furnas 1965: 122).

If we look at these hyperbolic statements in their historical context, we find that alcohol was not the only thing the new North American giant was out to reform. Tyrrell (2010) notes that the connections between the United States and Britain and northern Europe became more immediate than ever before by the invention of the telegraph and the laying of the transatlantic cable in 1866 (Tyrrell 2010:15). Some of the messages passing over those lines involved the exchange of social and moral ideals and plans for international conferences in furtherance of the agenda of moral reform. The forces supporting prohibition in the United States wanted, in addition to prohibiting alcoholic beverages, to curtail all forms of sex trade and to convert large segments of the world's population to their brand of Christian Protestant religion. Noted missionaries, including the Leitch siblings, contributed to reformist perspective by expressing their disgust with the lifestyle patterns seen in Paris in 1879 (Tyrrell 2010:26). Increasing ease of travel and communication did not simply familiarize travelers with how people in other countries lived; it whetted American missionaries' appetites for reforming the rest of the world (an objective that has hardly fallen by the wayside over time). The communication and travel advances of the 19th century gave the American missionaries reach that they never had before, and soon they dreamed dreams of a Christian, morally pure World Society. Another feature of the circulation that had become open and general was the improved accessibility of colonial holdings of the British Empire in Africa and Asia.

In a cultural context where "carry the white man's burden" had become something of a mantra, internationalism became highly fashionable by the late 1800s. Reformers envisioned a world in which peace, purity, and moral rectitude flourished, and the venal and corrupt were vanquished. To some Europeans, the linguistic vehicle for this world reform would be the synthetic "universal language," Esperanto, which began as a movement in the 1870s. In 1905, an international conference on Esperanto convened, but despite great enthusiasm among its advocates, the language never caught on (Tyrrell 2010:19). Linguistics as a discipline was at that time not very well developed, nor was the anthropological perspective on language as an integral part of culture. The emergence of Esperanto illustrates the naiveté and superficiality of the internationalist thinking that dominated the late 1800s. Apparently, the developers of Esperanto believed, as did Christian missionaries, that whenever benighted people encountered their superior language (and/or religious) system, they would naturally discard their own inferior system in favor of the superior one. A basic lesson of applied anthropology, however, is that people are not cultural blank slates upon which the inspired can inscribe their particular version of uplift and moral improvement.

The presumption of the movement of confident Westernization seems stunningly chauvinistic and racist, by present day standards—and entirely blind to the role Western imperialism was playing in the disruption of the world's peoples and diverse ways of life—but at the time, given the relative plenty enjoyed by Americans and Northwest Europeans (as a result of imperialism), it seemed not just logical, but altruistically beneficent to bring "superior" systems of belief, production, and morality to people who (they thought) had no knowledge of the "right" way to do things. All of this evangelistic/internationalistic attitude placed drinking in a category of behavior that, if its benighted practitioners could be convinced to "come to their senses," could be stamped out entirely. Unfortunately for the prohibitionists, none had the knowledge, wisdom, or cross-cultural perspective to recognize that their reformist plans were doomed. Instead of achieving world uplift, the prohibitionists' movement gathered enough impetus to send an entire nation into an immense and ultimately disastrous dead-end experiment.

We alluded earlier in this chapter to the role of women in the prohibitionist movement. The status of women in North America and Northwest Europe during the 19th century constituted an important factor in the formation and actions of women's groups that supported the temperance movement. In parallel to the development of women's organizations to promote temperance, women in the United Kingdom and the United States were preparing a campaign to allow women to vote in elections. The sensibilities that empowered women to react in opposition to the ways in which they presumed alcohol consumption disrupted their households were not very different from the ones that bridled at women's lack of suffrage. Indeed, seeing the adverse effect of heavy drinking on men, and what this said about their characters, may well have led some women to question the right of men to have a right that women lacked. Given the political context of the two movements and their parallels, it is hardly surprising that the Woman's Christian Temperance Union (WCTU), ultimately the most powerful of the women's organizations that supported prohibition, would engage energetically and successfully in politics (Tyrrell 1991:6). As their reach extended beyond the borders of the United States, it became necessary to establish a World Woman's Christian Temperance Union (WWCTU), an example of the internationalist intentions of would-be reformers based in the United States. As the WCTU and the WWCTU grew, they became increasingly powerful politically, and this power enabled the eventual ratification of Amendment 18 in 1919. Any politician interested in remaining incumbent between 1910 and 1930 found himself with the prospect of an electorate about to double in size, and a salient issue of concern for the new half of the electorate was prohibition. In the interest of self-preservation, that politician would seriously consider ratification of prohibition, regardless of his personal habits, beliefs, or proclivities. According to this interpretation, prohibition of alcoholic beverages was ratified in the United States as a direct consequence of the florescence of women's consciousness. Unfortunately, in that particular social context, the internationalist and chauvinistic ideas driving that consciousness helped launch a disaster.

In the course of constructing this disaster the prohibition movement succeeded in categorizing all of their fellow Americans as potential alcoholics, a line of thinking that played out similarly in the policies formed regarding other varieties of potentially addictive drugs. Whether the debate involved opioids, cannabis, or cocaine, the political rhetoric inevitably contained dire warnings about the drug equivalent of the "fatal glass of beer"; a mere taste could lead to a life of sin and perdition. The official stance assumed by the United States today seems to reflect a collective amnesia with regard to the first prohibition, as society's leaders persist, despite a track record of failure, in pursuing another prohibition. Organizations advocating the abolition of international opium trade began to form in the United States while the alcohol prohibition movement was gaining velocity (Blackman 2004:9). They would have a distinct influence on the legal status of opioids and other drugs in the years to come. In the succeeding chapters, we address these interpretations of human drug-using behavior and analyze their validity in terms of our direct field experience in studying drug use.

CHAPTER FOUR

Imagine That: Drug Users and Literature

The human history of culturally shaped material expression is ancient, with early examples being preserved as cave art, petroglyphs, and earth figures dating to the Upper Paleolithic period. In the course of human history, systematic recordkeeping in the form of inscription on a medium surpassed the spoken word as a culturally constituted mechanism to crystalize the memory of the flow of goods, events, and figures while facilitating the maintenance of the political-economic structure and inequality in human society. As writing came to inscribe human experience and the activities of living, it became a cross-cultural multivocal record of human involvement with psychotropic drugs and their impact on the human experience. This chapter examines this record historically exploring various literatures as a means of assessing patterns, themes, and attitudes that express the social construction of drugs and drug users in human society. Given the enormity of the human oeuvre, this review is selective, beginning with early religious writing and focusing especially on well-known works of fiction and authors whose writings and lives have included more than just a passing encounter with drugs. The objective is not to be exhaustive but sufficient to touch on key themes in the literary construction of the drug user and the role of drugs in literary production, including examples that at times seem to run counter to the broader arguments of the book (and why these were produced). At the same time, dark images of drug use, and woeful accounts of the adverse impacts of drugs on the lives (including as causes of death) of many writers, can be seen to support conventional attitudes about drug use and to reinforce acts of Othering and images of uselessness.

THE DEEPEST ROOTS OF DRUGS IN LITERATURE

Throughout recorded history, in many different cultural contexts, there have been inscribed local descriptions of people using drugs, often to the detriment of themselves and others, including classic works like the *Gilgamesh Epic*, the Vedas, the Torah, *The Rubaiyat*, and the writings of Homer.

The Social Value of Drug Addicts: The Uses of the Useless, by Merrill Singer and J. Bryan Page, 88–120.

These early written sources offer descriptions of states of intoxication and their consequences, including the basic theme that excess consumption damages the consumer of drugs. Yet that is not the sum total of their message, as drug use as a normal part of life is also a theme of ancient (as well as new) writing.

Gilgamesh is the best known of the ancient Mesopotamian heroes described in the *Gilgamesh Epic,* a collection of 12 incomplete Akkadian-language cuniform tablets dating to 3,000 years in the past. The tablets were discovered by archeologists in the remains of the library of Assyrian king Ashurbanipal near the modern city of Mosul in 1840. It is assumed that the Gilgamesh told of in the tablets was the ruler of Uruk (after which the country of Iraq is named) in southern Mesopotamia during the first half of the 3rd millennium BCE, although in the epic Gilgamesh is described is a demigod of superhuman strength and intense emotions. Although there is not extensive reference to alcohol in the tablets, it is mentioned as a normal part of life (Mitchell 2004).

The Vedas (which means knowledge or sacred teachings) are ancient Hindu texts, the oldest of which, the Rig Veda, was composed about 1500 BCE. There are three additional Vedas: the Sama Veda, Yajur Veda, and the Atharva-Veda. All are written in archaic Sanskrit and contain hymns, incantations, and rituals (e.g., how to make sacrificial offerings to the gods, the devas). In addition to being among the most ancient surviving religious texts, they offer a view of everyday life in India several thousand years ago. The Vedas are the work of the Aryans who came south to occupy the Indus Valley about 3,500 years ago. Among the gods of the Hindu pantheon is Soma, who was connected with an intoxicating plant-based drink used in Vedic rituals. In the Rig Veda there many hymns praising its energizing abilities. The hymns refer to the plant from which the juice is extracted to make soma as "God for Gods." Consuming soma, a libation of both the gods and humans, it is suggested in the Rig Veda, confers immortality. The actual plant in question, which is described as growing in the mountains, having long stalks, and a yellowish color, is unknown today, although some researchers favor a species of Ephedra, possibly *Ephedra sinica.* In his book "Food of the Gods," ethnobotanist and philosopher (and drug experimenter) Terence McKenna (1992) (who was introduced to the literary world of drug use through the writings of Aldous Huxley) suggested that a likely candidate for soma is the mushroom *Psilocybe cubensis,* a hallucinogenic mushroom. This mushroom can be found growing on cow dung in India. McKenna pointed out that the Rig Veda refers to the cow as the embodiment of soma.

The Vedas indicate that the soma drink was prepared by priests, who pounded the plants with stones to access its juices. These were collected and filtered through lamb's wool, and then mixed with other ingredients (such as milk) before it was drunk. The texts describing its effects (especially bringing "the light") suggest hallucinogenic properties. In addition soma is said to enhance alertness and awareness. Notably, more recent writers like William S. Burroughs and Aldous Huxley (see below) have used soma in their books, with Burroughs using it to label a form of opium said to have been in use in ancient India, while in Huxley's *Brave New World* it is presented as a drug consumed by people to quiet anxiety and adverse emotion.

The Torah, or so-called Old Testament, mentions various kinds of drug use among the ancient Hebrews. One of these drugs is derived from the mandrake plant, a member of the nightshades family, which is known to have psychoactive properties. The sources of this capacity are several potent hallucinogenic alkaloids, such as atropine, scopolamine, and apoatropine. Mandrake is mentioned in Genesis 30:14–16 and in Song of Solomon 7:13.

Moreover, consuming wine was a normal part of everyday life among the ancient Hebrews and intoxication was apparently not uncommon. Noah, for example, planted a vineyard and upon harvesting his fruit got quite drunk. Overall the Torah is somewhat ambivalent toward alcohol consumption, describing wine, on the one hand, as both a gift from God (needed in various rituals), a medicinal drink, and a source of jollity, and, on the other, as a cause of sinful behavior. In addition to wine, the Torah refers to strong drink, which, because of a lack distillation among the ancient Hebrews may have referred to various forms of beer.

Beyond these drugs, as anthropologist Vera Rubin (1975) noted, various references to marihuana can be found in the Torah. According to Sula Benet (1975), a Polish etymologist who was affiliated with the Institute of Anthropological Sciences in Warsaw, "In the original Hebrew text of the Old Testament there are allusions to hemp, both as incense, which was an integral part of religious celebration, and as an intoxicant." Notably, anthropologist Weston La Barre (1975), noted for his study of peyote use in the Native American Church, referred to various biblical references in an essay on marihuana. For example, Exodus 30:23 is interpreted by some scholars as including a possible reference to marihuana.

The Rubáiyát of Omar Khayyám is the title used by translator Edward FitzGerald (2011) for a selection of ancient Persian poems. The title refers to the use of a quatrain pattern in the poems (a ruba'i being a two-line stanza with two parts). The original author of the poems lived from 1048 to 1131, making *The Rubáiyát,* with its references to wine, a window on attitudes about drinking from times long past.

Exemplary of this attitude about wine are these quatrains:

> Did God set grapes a-growing, do you think,
> And at the same time make it sin to drink?
> Give thanks to Him who foreordained it thus—
> Surely He loves to hear the glasses clink!
> I desire a little ruby wine and a book of verses,
> Just enough to keep me alive, and half a loaf is needful;
> And then, that I and thou should sit in a desolate place
> Is better than the kingdom of a sultan.
> In spring if a houri [virgin in paradise]-like sweetheart
> Gives me a cup of wine on the edge of a green cornfield,
> Though to the vulgar this would be blasphemy,
> If I mentioned any other Paradise, I'd be worse than a dog.

If these translations are correct and they are read literally (some commentators view the text as symbolic expression of Sufi mystical understandings of the divine rather than early attitudes and pleasures) it would seem that wine is held to be a normal part of life, indeed one of life's enrichments, and thus is approved by a benevolent god. Overindulgence is not addressed but rather drinking as a pathway to early enjoyment.

Homer, the ancient Greek poet, is best known for his *Illiad* and the *Odyssey,* which had a sweeping impact on the subsequent history of Western literature. While it remains uncertain, Homer is believed to have lived somewhere in the 7th or 8th centuries BCE. From his work, it is evident that Homer was well aware of intoxication, drug-related supernatural inspiration, and hallucinogenic visionary experiences, as these appear as consistent themes in his work. For example, in the *Odyssey,* he describes a group of people, known as the Lotus-Eaters, who spent their days getting high and forgetting about routine responsibilities and life's troubles. (Hill 2008). The source of their altered awareness was the seductive honey-sweet fruit of the lotus plant, which stifled any motivation they might have to do anything else but get high and provided them with the experience of absentminded bliss. In the text, Odysseus tells of his efforts to rescue some of his soldiers who have encountered the temptations of the Lotus-Eaters' approach to life. The plant made the solders feel good enough to lay down their weapons, reject warrior Greek culture, and spend their days consuming the narcotic lotus. This episode suggests an underlying tension that might have existed in Greek society at the time of Homer between a celebration of marshal virtue and the violence of the battlefield, on the one side, and those who came to object to endless conflict and its alarming costs, on the other. At the same time, it reveals a degree of ambivalence about drug use, which offers an escape from life's burdens and demands, but leads to stuporous indolence.

Through these brief glimpses into the literary past, it is possible to see that the harsh condemnatory attitudes that were later to emerge, as well as the categorization of the drug user as a distinct class of dangerous Others were not part of earlier thinking and writing about those for whom drug use is a pivotal element in their life course. The drug user as a useless and threatening boogey man was constructed over time in a world of changing social structures and relationships, a process in which literature plays a complex and even contradictory part.

DRUG USERS AS WRITERS AND WRITINGS ABOUT DRUG USERS

In 2000, famed horror writer Stephen King, author of a long series of short stories and best-selling novels, including *Carrie, The Shining, Misery,* and *The Green Mile,* and a bestselling author of the 20th century, remarked during an interview, "With cocaine, one snort, and it just owned my body and soul.... Cocaine was my on-switch, and it seemed like a really good energizing drug. You try some and think, 'Wow why haven't I been taking this for years?'" (quoted in Rogak 2010:96). In these words, King expressed his initial experience with cocaine, although his use of other drugs had begun years earlier. Like many well-known (e.g., John Keats, Ernest Hemmingway, James Baldwin, Tennessee Williams, Marcel Proust, Jean Cocteau, Dorothy Parker, William Faulkner, and Mary Karr) and many lesser known authors, King's personal life was filled with the use of drugs for many years.

For some authors, personal drug use provides the experience and imagery that fills their stories, poems, and other literary production. Since Thomas de Quincey's 1822 confessions of opium consumption, literary readers have been exposed to profuse representations of drug use, its benefits and dangers, its social worlds, and place in relationships through printed words. The following section of this chapter examines the application of mind-altered experiences to the process of creative writing generally and creative writing that specifically incorporates descriptions, scenes, praises, and warnings about drug use.

MY LIFE ON DRUGS

Drugs, for shorter or longer periods, have been a significant element in the lives of many authors, and many have written about it in autobiographical works. For some, this has been a sublime experience, for others a tragic one, although most heavily drug-involved writers have experienced both the heaven and hell of drug consumption.

In the case of already-mentioned Stephen King, much of the 1980s was spent on a protracted drug and alcohol binge that so impacted his memory that even today he cannot recall working on the numerous books he produced during that period. King admitted that drugs helped him cope with the dreadful unhappiness that haunted him since his childhood in Portland, Maine, after the Second World War. King's father abandoned the family when he was two and he long feared his mother, who was forced to take various menial jobs, would do the same. Plagued by nightmares, as a child King's imagination was filled with grisly images of his mother laid out in a coffin and himself swinging from a gallows, with crows pecking out his eyes. His days were driven by multiple fearful and destructive anxieties which included a gnawing sense that he would be sucked down the toilet, an inescapable preoccupation with death, and macabre thoughts about body deformities. Eventually, King realized that one way he could deal with his burdensome angst was by writing stories about them, based on the idiosyncratic belief that if he could write about something frightening it would not happen. While an English student at the University of Maine, he found that drugs like marihuana, amphetamine, alcohol, and LSD also were useful in controlling his many anxieties.

After graduation, married with two children and working as a high-school teacher, King, aspiring to be an author, encountered growing frustration in trying to get his stories and novels published. When his mother died in 1973, he fell into a deep depression that hung on even as his first book *Carrie* was published, an event that earned him a sizeable royalty and allowed him to become a full-time writer. Still saddled with dark thoughts, he began to drink and smoke heavily, and was introduced to cocaine, which was readily available at the Hollywood parties he attended as *Carrie* and *The Shining* were made into movies toward the end of the 1970s. All of these drugs, he felt, helped drive him through intense late-night writing marathons, and cope with his newly acquired fears of snakes, rats, and the number 13. He came to believe that he would be unable to write if he was not under the influence powerful chemicals.

In *On Writing, A Memoir of The Craft* (King 2000), a biographical essay, King wrote about his brother David who was struck by a drunk driver and almost died. He also reported on his drug and alcohol addiction explaining that he got drunk for the first time in 1966 during a senior class trip to Washington. In the mid-1980s King wrote *Misery*, the title of which, and its exploration of entrapment, he revealed, described his state of mind at the time because of his drug use. In 1986, he wrote *The Tommyknockers*, commonly working until late into the night with his heart pounding and cotton swabs wedged in his nose to stop the bleeding caused by snorting abundant quantities of cocaine. Notably, *The Tommyknockers* was about alien beings from whom humans could get super energy at the price of their souls. King explained that while he did not intend the book's theme to be a metaphor for his own relationship with drugs and alcohol, his subconscious probably did. King also reported that Jack Torrance, the recovering alcoholic character in his book *The Shining*, was modeled on his memories of his own alcoholic father. In the novel, the character Torrance thinks about drinking all the time and eventually gets drunk and goes on a murderous rampage. Throughout the book, alcoholism is linked to dysfunctional families, domestic abuse, and cycles of family violence. Some reviewers have interpreted *The Shining* as a temperance narrative that argues against alcohol consumption.

Ultimately, in his own life, King reached the point that he was spending most of his days high while suffering from blackouts from the drugs he consumed. Confronted by his wife and family about his self-destructiveness, he began to change his ways, only to be thrust into a period of painful writer's block. As he emerged from the latter, his stories lost some of their haunted intensity but King has remained a highly successful and well-published author.

King's life has been characterized by a troublesome contradiction: drugs were part of the fuel that drove him to literary success but also the toxin that almost destroyed his life. In this, among literary authors, King is not alone. Indeed, five of the nine Americans to win the Nobel Prize for Literature had significant alcohol-related problems, a group that includes Sinclair Lewis (1930), Eugene O'Neill (1936), William Faulkner (1949), Ernest Hemingway (1954), and John Steinbeck (1962). Indeed, the idea that drugs are a vital part of the writing experience, fueling creativity and unchaining the writer's imagination, has had a life of its own among both successful and would-be writers. This notion is sharply disputed by others. Iain Smith, psychiatrist and addiction expert from Scotland, argues instead that

The reason why this myth is so powerful is the allure of the substances, and the fact that many artists need drugs to cope with their emotions. Artists are, in general, more emotional people.... [But w]hen you try and capture the experiences [triggered by drugs] they are often nonsense. These drugs often wipe your memory, so it's hard to remember how you were in that state of mind (quoted in Van Radowitz 2010).

Without question, for some well-known authors, alcohol destroyed both their literary ability and their life. F. Scott Fitzgerald, for example, gained success as a writer while in his early 20s, selling stories about life during the Roaring Twenties that earned him access to an immoderate lifestyle characterized by frequent parties and regular drinking. While writing his most celebrated novel, *The Great Gatsby* (Fitzgerald 1993), he was able to refrain from drinking. But the success of this work led to considerable social pressure to produce a follow-up best seller. Regular drinking, however, made it difficult for him to focus on a novel-length project. He focused instead on writing short stories that he could sell for quick access to cash. By the late 1920s, Fitzgerald began to see alcohol as necessary for his writing, the energy fueling his artistic facilities. In 1931, he moved to Hollywood to start up a career as a screen writer. But his drunken behavior during Hollywood parties led him to being fired. By his 40th birthday, he had hit bottom and attempted suicide by drinking a bottle of morphine. In the last years of his life, Fitzgerald experienced worsening symptoms related to alcohol consumption, and he died of a heart attack at the age of 44.

Another noteworthy example of an author's rocky encounter with alcohol is that of John Sutherland, a professor of English literature in England, a self-confessed "recovering drunk" and author of *Last Drink to LA* (Sutherland 2001). In this book, Sutherland relays his own struggles with alcohol and his experiences in Alcoholics Anonymous. Listening to his fellow AA members share their life stories and long-term relationships with "booze," he came to believe that the one thing about alcohol addiction is that it makes you good at is storytelling, although most the stories he heard at AA meetings he believed to be exaggerated and self-serving. To the degree that alcohol lubricates storytelling capacity, it is perhaps not surprising how frequently heavy and problematic drinking is found among writers. What drives some people to write—deep personal suffering—may also drive them to drink. The experience of alcohol's effects, in turn, finds its way into what they write, how they write, and may in time join the causes of why they write or fail to write.

A somewhat muddied and much earlier case is that of Edgar Allen Poe, a famed writer of the horror genre who certainly used drugs (in particular, alcohol) and wrote about drug-using characters. But the full impact of drugs on his life has remained an issue of dispute for over one hundred years. Also mysterious are the conditions of Poe's death and the role of drugs in his demise. Based on various sources of information, it is commonly concluded that Poe was an alcoholic. On its website, the partisan Edger Allan Poe Society of Baltimore notes (2009),

> Certainly, Poe drank and often drank more than was good for him, even after he had promised himself to stay away from alcohol. It also seems likely that Poe's father (David Poe Jr.) and brother (Henry Poe) were hard-core drinkers.

Still the society asserts that Poe's depictions of drug use were not autobiographical but only served as a literary device. Poe's use of drugs, the Society maintains, was sporadic and not a major force in this literary career. Yet Poe is known to have been dismissed from his job at the *Southern Literary Messenger* in the mid-1830s because of alcoholism and to have increased his drinking and drug use after the death of his young wife. Interestingly, 147 years after his death, doctors at the University of Maryland Medical Center concluded that Poe died of rabies and not from the complications of alcoholism (as was long asserted by some literary historians). This conclusion was based on a medical review of Poe's condition in the hospital several days before his death, most prominently suggested by the fact that he had trouble drinking water and slipped in and out of consciousness and lucidity during this period (which is characteristic of rabies and not alcoholism).

Whatever Poe's personal practices, it is undeniable that characters he created used drugs. Exemplary is the short story "Lady Ligeia," (1838) in which the narrator is presented as smoking opium while sitting with his dead wife's corpse overnight. While under the influence, he hallucinates that his long lost love, Lady Ligeia (a woman the narrator describes as having the radiance of an opium dream), has come back from the dead and taken possession of the lifeless body of his deceased wife. Uniting elements like the macabre, mental illness, and the use of mind-altering drugs, Poe achieved a renowned place in the pantheon of the American literati. In doing so, he communicated a particularly dark message about drug use that nonetheless harmonizes with other such cultural assertions.

WRITING UNDER THE INFLUENCE

A notably large number of well-known and celebrated literary contributions were composed under the influence of mind-altering drugs. Philosopher and writer Sadie Plant (1999:265–266) has suggested in her fast-paced, fact-filled, but meandering cultural history of drug use, that the methodology in this approach to composition,

> is to plunge into a world where nothing is as simple or as stable as it seems. Everything about it shimmers and mutates as you try to hold its gaze. Facts and figures dance around each other; lines of inquiry scatter like expensive dust.

The challenges of writing with high doses of psychotropics "on board," as (Kimiya 2000) emphasizes stem from the fact that

> As anyone who has ever tried to write anything after partaking of psychoactive substances knows, altered states of consciousness go into words the way a tsunami goes into a squirt gun. Your synapses may be firing like Gatling guns, your mind may be soaring through the empyrean, but what you succeed in getting down on paper are incoherent gestures, endless digressions and fragments of fragments.

And yet, many pages have been filled, and often successfully so, by writers following the ingestion of a variety of drugs, often in combination. In 1797, for example, the influential Romantic poet and literary critic Samuel Taylor Coleridge wrote the symbolic poem "Kubla Khan or A Vision in a Dream" (which is believed to be a poem about poetry) while taking the patented narcotic drug laudanum (to treat anxiety and depression). Images for the never-finished poem had their origin in a drug-induced dream that followed Coleridge's reading the book *Purchas, His Pilgrimage, or Relations of the World and Religions Observed in All Ages and Places Discovered, from the Creation to the Present* that briefly described Xanadu, the summer palace of the Mongol ruler and Emperor of China Kublai Khan. The poem, guided by Coleridge's conviction that writing should pull the reader into willing suspension of disbelief in things our rational minds would otherwise reject, was facilitated by opium ingestion to allow Coleridge "to explore life on the line between illusion and truth [while making] it difficult for him to reassert the difference between the two" (Plant 1999:22). During the later years of his life it is believed that Coleridge consumed as much as two quarts of laudanum—an alcoholic herbal preparation containing approximately 10% powdered opium by weight—a week. Coleridge joined the ranks of writers who struggle with addiction for many years; in Coleridge's case unsuccessfully so, and he died a victim of his drug use in 1834 at the age of 61. Even before he succumbed to its powers, Coleridge suffered continually from a gut-wrenching sense of guilt about being a user, condemning himself repeatedly in letters, lamenting

> ingratitude to my maker for the wasted Talents; ingratitude to so many of my friends who have loved me I know not why; of barbarous neglect of my family ... I have in this one dirty business of Laudanum a hundred times deceived, tricked, nay, actually and consciously *lied*—And yet all these vices are so opposite to my nature, that but for this *free-agency-annihilating Poison,* I verily believe that I should have suffered myself to be cut in pieces rather than have committed any one of them (Ingram 1998:223).

Scottish writer Robert Louis Stevenson's drug of choice was cocaine. It is alleged that he wrote his famous *The Strange Case of Dr Jekyll and Mr Hyde* (1886) during a six-day cocaine binge (although this is disputed by some literary historians). He used cocaine to treat his tuberculosis. The novella is about a London lawyer named Gabriel John Utterson who investigates the strange relationship of his old friend Dr Henry Jekyll to the evil figure known as Edward Hyde (in a case of dissociative identity disorder), a story that became one of Stevenson's best sellers. His wife Fanny said of the novella's writing: "That an invalid in my husband's condition performed the manual labour alone seems incredible. He was suffering from continual haemorrhages and hardly allowed to speak, his conversation carried on by means of a slate and pencil." (quoted in Ezard 2000). But finish he did. He even went on to write *In the South Seas,* (1896) which constitutes a strong piece of lay ethnography based on Stevenson's travels to various Pacific islands.

In the short book, Stevenson tells the tale of a genteel and refined aristocrat who is consumed by the dark power of an unknown chemical addiction, which in Mathiasen's (2009) view, expresses a moralistic attitude toward addiction. One likely suspect for the drug that ravages Dr Jekyll and unleashes the beast within him, Mr. Hyde, is opium, which, as discussed below, was well-known from the opium dens that sprang up around London during the Victorian era in which Stevenson lived (Wright 1994). Additionally, there is Stevenson's (1886:70) description of the drug's effects spoken by Dr Jekyll: "The most racking pangs succeeded: a grinding in the bones, deadly nausea, and a horror

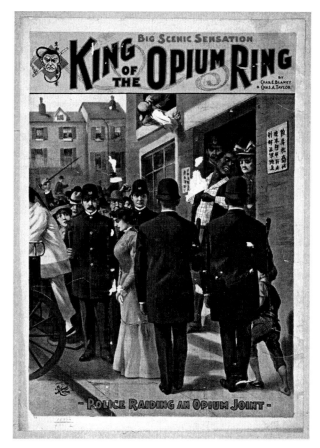

Police raid on London opium joint

of the spirit that cannot be exceeded at the hour of birth or death. Then these agonies began to swiftly subside, and I came to myself as out of great sickness." Unable to bear the duality of his tortured drug-dependent existence, Dr Jekyll commits suicide, a final moral warning about the evils of psychoactive drugs.

Acclaimed Victorian poet Elizabeth Barrett Browning began the use of laudanum while still a teenager as a treatment for various nervous disorders (known during the patriarchal era of her life as hysteria, a consequence of having debilitating female hormones). Also part of her treatment, which she called her elixir, especially for insomnia and what she described in a letter to her husband as "continual aching sense of weakness" (quoted in Aiken 2012) were opium and morphine mixed with ether. These she praised for their tranquilizing effect and viewed as necessary for her poetic efforts. In her letters, Browning described intense drug-sustained writing sessions and productivity: "I am in a fit of writing—could write all day and night—& long to live by myself for 3 months in a forest of chestnuts and cedars in an hourly succession of poetical paragraphs and morphine draughts" (quoted in Aiken 20, 2011). As her dependence on drugs became known in literary circles, American poet Julia Ward Howe, author of "The Battle Hymn of the Republic," accused her of relying on opium as her primary source of poetic imagination. While this accusation upset her, she admitted to her husband that the charge "was perfectly true, so far, that life is necessary to writing, & that I should not be alive except by help of my morphine" (quoted in Foxcroft 2007:48). Despite her attachment to drugs, Browning was aware that others might view her behavior as degenerate and was thus concerned that it be known that her drug use was medicinal and hence respectable in the eyes of society. In another letter to her husband she more playfully asked, "Can I be as good for you as morphine is for me. I wonder, even at the cost of being as bad also?" Her always protective husband's romantic response: "May I call you my morphine?" (quoted in Foxcroft 2007:46). Following two miscarriages, Browning cut back the extent of her drug use, fearful that drugs might have poisoned her unborn children. Eventually, she gave birth to a son when she was forty-three.

Celebrated American science-fiction writer Philip K. Dick, author of numerous novels as well as various essays and short stories, used the amphetamine-like drug semoxydrine as well as various hallucinogens to inspire many of his works. Best known of his collected works were the novels *Do Androids Dream of Electric Sheep? Time Out Of Joint, The Three Stigmata of Palmer Eldritch,* and the Hugo-award winning *The Man In The High Castle.* Despite his over productivity, Dick had a chaotic personal life, with five marriages and rotating bouts of ability and inability to produce. Moreover, he was weighted down by what he experienced as direct encounters with the divine. The final years of Dick's life were haunted by a visitation from God, or God-like being. Dick spent a number of years writing journals regarding this asserted visitation and his interpretations of the event. His last novels all deal in some way with the being in his visions, especially *Valis,* in which the title character is an extraterrestrial God-like machine that contacts a schizophrenic and possibly drug-addicted science fiction writer named Philip K. Dick. Despite his award-winning novels and broad acclaim, Dick was never financially successful. Toward the very end of his life, however, he achieved a degree of financial stability, in part from the money he received from the producers of *Blade Runner* for the rights to his novel *Do Androids Dream of Electric Sheep?*

Iconic Beat Generation writer Jean Louis (Jack) Kerouac produced the initial draft of his legendary and impulsive *On the Road* in less than three weeks. The "spontaneous prose" method (Kerouac's term) that characterized his writing style was shaped in no small measure by his consumption of drugs while at his writing desk. In his master's thesis on Kreouac, Eric Izant (2008) argued that the altered states of consciousness produced by Kerouac's drug use should be considered in conjunction with historical, cultural, and biographical factors in tracing the evolution of Kerouac's creativity. As a leading member of the Beat Generation, Kerouac regularly used drugs as both social expression of rebellion against mainstream 1950s American society and because of the belief that it offered artistic insight. The latter idea has a long tradition among writers and other artists who come to view drugs as modern-day muses and accessible chemical gateways to a transcendental realm of visionary truth. Kerouac, who believed writing in English had lost its potential for true communication because the art had become ossified in rigid forms of proper grammar and sentence construction, sought a prose style that would allow the highest levels of authenticity in expressions of human experience and emotion. Kerouac used drugs like amphetamine (in the form of Benzedrine), marihuana, and alcohol, each of which offered their own altered perception, to achieve new frames of consciousness, and then recreated and expressed these altered states through his writing. The first of these drugs fueled Kerouac's legendary typing marathons, allowing him to not only expeditiously write *On the Road* in a few weeks but works like *The Subterraneans* in three days.

The core features of Kerouac's prose style involved a de-emphasis on revision, limited punctuation, and the use of long-flowing sentences. He also sought to share subjective experiences truthfully, an ability he believed was aided by the use of marihuana. Marihuana also provided a dream-like quality to Kerouac's texts. Later, he wrote *Desolation Angel's* while sober, suggesting that Kerouac's belief that drugs were a necessity for his style may not have been completely true. During the latter part of his career, Kerouac turned to alcohol, which he consumed prodigiously during the writing of *Big Sur* and *Vanity of Duluoz*. These later works were characterized by a less rebellious style that appears to have been influenced by rampant alcohol abuse. He died at the age of 47 (1969) due to internal bleeding caused by alcohol abuse, resulting in his life, if not his art, providing support for the threats of drug use.

WRITING OF THE EXPERIENCE

Beyond writing books under the experience of drugs, authors also have written them about the experience of drugs. Beginning with Thomas de Quincey, who has been mentioned in previous chapters, autobiographical texts about drug use and its impact on the writers' lives have communicated quite contrasting messages, both positive and negative about life on drugs. De Quincey's influential autobiographical account of his addiction to opium, entitled *Confessions of an English Opium Eater* was published in 1822. Feldman and Aldrich (1990) credit de Quincey as being the first writer to produce a book-length work that could fairly be called a "drug ethnography." Having first taken opium to relieve a prolonged headache, de Quincey went on to use the drug for ten years because of the "artificial state of pleasure" that it brought him. Although an adventurer and not a trained social scientist, de Quincey, who spent a number of years living among the urban poor, was a keen observer of the significant upsurge in opium and alcohol use in the working-class districts of London during the Industrial Revolution. "Happiness might now be bought for a penny," he wrote, "and carried in the waistcoat pocket; portable ecstasies might be had *corked* up in a pint bottle; and peace of mind could be sent down in gallons by the mail pouch" (de Quincey 1822:44). As Plant (1999:8) points out, "Opium grew in popularity in the late eighteenth century, as the first steam engines sputtered to life and the first great factories were built." De Quincey also was interested in drug use among prominent individuals, those whose lives were made comfortable by the rise of industrialization, such as intellectuals like the poet Samuel Taylor Coleridge. In his book, de Quincey recorded his personal experiences with and observations of opium use across social classes. Unlike in Asia where it was smoked, the opium users observed by de Quincy drank it in liquid form, a practice that continued until the introduction of the hypodermic needle. As part of his assessment of the experience of opium, he (de Quincey 1822:55) contrasted it with drinking wine, saying:

> [T]he main distinction [between wine and opium] lies in this, that whereas wine disorders the mental faculties, opium, on the contrary ... introduces amongst them the most exquisite order, legislation, and harmony.... Wine unsettles and clouds the judgment, ... opium, on the contrary, communicates serenity and equipoise to all the faculties, active or passive: and with respect to the temper and moral feelings in general, it gives simply that sort of vital warmth which is approved by the judgment.

The book brought him almost overnight celebrity and formed the template for many writers who attempted to follow in de Quincey's staggering footsteps.

One of those was Charles Baudelaire, a French poet, art critic and translator (e.g., of Edgar Allan Poe) and the publisher of a popular French translation of de Quincey's book entitled "Les paradis artificiels." Baudelaire is also credited with coining the term "modernity" to describe life in the metropolis and the role of art in capturing that experience. Baudelaire was a member of the Club de Hachichins (Hashish Club), which met in Paris between 1844 and 1849 and included among its distinguished membership individuals like Alexandre Dumas, Honoré de Balzac, Victor Hugo, Jacques-Joseph Moreau, and Eugène Delacroix. The club was dedicated to exploring drug-induced experiences, especially hashish. Exploration of this sort was common in elite intellectual, scientific, and literary circles. The club convened monthly séances at the Hôtel Pimodan to discuss and partake of their drug of choice.

As his own contribution to the "drug experience" genre, Baudelaire wrote extensively in essays about using hashish, which reflect, as Plant (1999:39) comments, included "swings between love and hatred." In his view, expressed in The Poem of Hashish (2004 [original 1885]), "Among the drugs most efficient in creating what I call the artificial ideal ... the most convenient and the most handy are hashish and opium." Opium for Baudelaire as it was for Coleridge was laudanum, of which he was a long-time user. Yet, ultimately Baudelaire "condemned hashish as a means of circumventing the effort and time it takes to reap [great] rewards, a shortcut to paradise" (Plant 1999:39).

American author, journalist, and explorer Fitz Hugh Ludlow, who has been described as "America's first famous dope fiend" (Gross 1995), gained celebrity for his autobiographical work, "The Hasheesh Eater" (1857). Ludlow was born into a religious family in New York City, to sickly mother and ministerial father who was an active abolitionist involved in the Underground Railroad. Ludlow graduated from college in the years just before the start of the Civil War, having befriended during his college years an apothecary whose shop was the site of his introduction to various psychotropic drugs. Although he passed the bar, Ludlow selected a writing career rather than becoming a lawyer and quickly began publishing articles for various popular and well-read magazines of his day. From early on, many of his writing, including his first publication, "The Apocalypse of Hasheesh" (2009a [1856]), addressed hashish and opium use, drugs he used as part of the literary bohemian subculture of New York City centered at Pfaff's beer cellar on Broadway, a milieu that included Walt Whitman. Later, he would travel west to California and fall in with the literary coterie he found there, which at the time—prior to his rise to literary fame—counted Mark Twain among its members. Back in the East, Ludlow married Rosalie Osborne, whose mother had misgivings about the union given Ludlow's well-known involvement with drugs. He fathered several children, but died of tuberculosis at the age of 34.

In writing about hasheesh in his "Apocalypse" article, Ludlow (2009a) observed:

> The value of this experience to me consists in its having thrown open to my gaze many of those sublime avenues in the spiritual life, at whose gates the soul in its ordinary state is forever blindly groping, mystified, perplexed, yet earnest to the last in its search for that secret spring which, being touched, shall swing back the colossal barrier. In a single instant I have seen the vexed question of a lifetime settled, the mystery of some grand recondite process of mind laid bare, the last grim doubt that hung persistently on the sky of a sublime truth blown away.

Despite the intense and vivid sense of spiritual uplift, awakening to a deeper and fuller meaning of life, and the experience of "towering into sublimity," Ludlow's account of using hasheesh is counterbalanced by a palpable dark side.

> Upon my head, in a tremendous and ever-thickening cloud, came slowly down the guilt of all the ages past, and all the world to come; by a dreadful quickening, I beheld every atrocity and nameless crime coming up from all time on lines that centred in myself (Ludlow 2009a).

His book-length treatment, *The Hasheesh Eater,* was influenced by his reading of de Quincey's *Confessions of an English Opium Eater.* It was clear that he avoided writing about opium to avoid hostile comparison with de Quincey's work. In Plant's (1999:36) view, "there is little doubt that Ludlow was seduced by the drama of de Quincey's addiction." In his book, Ludlow further described the experience of altered consciousness through the use of Cannabis (specifically the resin from the flowers of the female plant) and the philosophical reflections it generated, including the terror of feeling overwhelmed by the drug.

> I could not doubt it. I was in the power of the hashesh influence. My first emotion was one of uncontrollable terror—a sense of getting something

which I did not bargain for. That moment I would have given all I had or hoped to have to be as I was three hours before (Ludlow 1857:20).

Despite this initial dread, Ludlow, who was just 21 years old when his book was published, proceeded to describe in florid detail the hallucinogenic expansion of space and time experienced under the influence, noting

One portion of me whirled unresistingly along the track of this tremendous experience, the other sat looking down from a height upon its double, observing, reasoning, and serenely weighing all the phenomena.... I dwelt in a marvelous inner world. I existed by turns in different places and various states of being (Ludlow 1857:23).

Ludlow came like other drug-using writers to believe that drug use was a boon to his creativity, although he also recognized that his pen could but poorly record the elaborate and changing hallucinatory visions experienced when he was high.

Although he could not overcome his own drug dependency, Ludlow, perhaps drawing on memories of his father's activism, became deeply committed to helping others struggling with addiction. This work was guided by his belief that the opium addict "is a proper subject, not for reproof, but for medical treatment" (Ludlow 2009b [1868]:379). One of his essays, "John Heathburn's Title" (1864), describes an opium and alcohol addict who is cured through the patience of a sympathetic physician using a substitution therapy composed of a Cannabis extract. It is based on Ludlow's own efforts in treating opium addicts that came to him seeking help. He also authored "Outlines of the Opium-Cure" (Ludlow 2009b) in which he described an elaborate therapeutic plan involving isolation in comfortable surroundings, baths and massages, nutritional diet, and diminishing administration of opium over a month's course. One of Ludlow's (1870) last published articles, written for the *New York Tribune,* also appears to have been prompted by his work with destitute opiate addicts. Entitled the "Homes for the Friendless," the essay advocated the establishment of homeless shelters for alcoholics and other drug addicts. The idea was warmly embraced by Tribune editor Horace Greeley.

English writer and satirist Aldous Huxley, best known for his celebrated book *Brave New World (1932),* also authored *The Doors of Perception* (1994), a work that inspired Jim Morrison's choice of his band's name and the drug-informed style of his music. In the vogue of Ludlow's most famous work,

Huxley provides a detailed account of his experience with the drug mescaline. Extracted from the Peyote cactus, mescaline induces hallucinations which Huxley found opened his mind and inspired him in his creative endeavors. Huxley's attraction to mescaline was rooted in his long-time interest in spiritualism. Huxley first heard of peyote use while learning about ceremonies of the Native American Church in New Mexico soon after coming to the United States from the United Kingdom in 1937. He also read about mescaline in an academic paper written by Humphry Osmond, a British psychiatrist working at Weyburn Mental Hospital, Saskatchewan in early 1952. Huxley wrote to Osmand indicating his desire to be an experimental subject in mescaline research. He hoped the drug would bring him closer to spiritual enlightenment. Osmond, although having some reluctance, agreed and traveled to California for this purpose. The drug was administered in the hills overlooking Hollywood. Subsequently, over a one-month period (after a three-week road trip around several national parks), Huxley wrote his famous drug book. He explained his motivation for taking mescaline as a hope to gain new insight into extraordinary states of mind and expected to see brightly colored fanciful landscapes. While this did not occur, Huxley stated that the drug changed his perception of the external world. After the book was published, and was rebuffed in some circles, Huxley wrote to Harold Raymond that he found it strange that when Hilaire Belloc and G. K. Chesterton wrote praises of alcohol they did not lose their standing as good Christians, but when someone suggests other paths to self-transcendence they are accused of being a drug addict and of being depraved (Murray 2003). Nonetheless, Huxley continued to use mind-altering drugs for the rest of his life and for a time befriended Timothy Leary with whom he shared an appreciation of the value of drug use. Notably, years later when stricken by cancer, and on his deathbed unable to speak any longer, Huxley wrote a request to his wife Laura for 100 μg of LSD, which she obliged.

Certainly a star of the "experience with drugs" genre was American novelist William Burroughs, who drew on his experience with opioids throughout his writing, especially in the books *Junkie* (1953) and *Naked Lunch* (1959). Burroughs penned the latter book in Morocco while under the influence of marihuana and an opium derivative called Eukodol (Townsend 2008). For many years, Burroughs kept his sexual orientation concealed, but with the publication of *Naked Lunch* he came out of the closet to become a recognized homosexual writer (and a controversial one, as he was tried for breaking US sodomy laws because of the content of the book). Burroughs attended Harvard University as an undergraduate and even had a brief try as a graduate student of anthropology at Harvard, and later a similarly short experience as a medical student in Vienna, Austria. Like Kerouac, with whom he once lived (he also lived in the same rundown rooming house in Paris as Alan Ginsberg, his lover Gregory Corso, and Peter Orlovsky), Burroughs was a member of the Beat Generation of writers. In fact, he and Kerouac wrote a novel together about an incident involving their failure to report a murder they knew of, but the two novice writers were unable to find a publisher (although the book was published many years later in 2008). It was during this time that Burroughs began using morphine, and he was soon addicted, and even later sold heroin in New York City to support his drug habit.

His experience in the international world of drugs (which for Burroughs included time spent in Mexico City, London, Paris, Berlin, the South American Amazon, and Tangier) provided semiautobiographical material for most of Burroughs's texts. His publications, in turn, provided needed cash to purchase drugs. At one point, Burroughs enrolled in a drug-treatment program in London, but soon relapsed (after writing a letter about his treatment experience to *The British Journal of Addictions* published in 1956). For a time, he even joined the Church of Scientology and initially claimed that their therapeutic system helped him, although he later had a falling out with the Scientologists that led to a sharp exchange of letters with members of the Church in *Rolling Stone Magazine* (Wills 2011).

Although his work was condemned by some as obscene (and he was prosecuted on these grounds in several states), his ultimate success as a writer is signified by his election to the American Academic and Institute of Arts and Letters, as well as being awarded the *Ordre des Arts et des Lettres* by France after publication of three experimental novels—The Soft Machine (1961), The Ticket that Exploded (1962), and Nova Express (1964)—that together have come to be known as *The Nova Trilogy*. In 1983, Burroughs was elected to the American Academy and Institute of Arts and Letters, and in 1984 was awarded. He died of a heart attack in Kansas in 1997.

The prodigious drug appetite of American journalist and author Hunter Stockton Thompson gained him recognition in the drug literature, especially for his 1972 book *Fear and Loathing in Las Vegas*. The book, which began as an assignment for *Sports Illustrated* to cover a desert motorcycle race, recounts a drug-drenched road-trip that he took to Sin City in 1971. The book, which opens with the attention-grabbing sentence: "We were somewhere around Barstow on the edge of the desert when the drugs began to take hold" (Thompson 1998:1). Thompson explains the drugs in question by explaining that he launched his trip (in both senses of the word) in possession of two bags of marihuana, 75 pellets of mescaline, five sheets of LSD, a salt shaker half full of cocaine, a pint of ether, some tequila, rum, and beer, and a diverse collection of pharmaceutical products characterized by multiple colors and brain effects. The book offers a heavily drug-shaped rumination on the failure of the 1960s counterculture movement as well as a healthy dose of Thompson's ire at the hypocrisy of American life. In the book, the narrator comments that Las Vegas "is not a good town for psychedelic drugs. Reality itself is too twisted" (Thompson 1998:47).

First serialized in *Rolling Stone,* a magazine with which Thompson had a long-time association, it was called "best book on the dope decade" by the *New York Times Book Review* (Woods 1972). In 1988, it was made into a movie starring Johnny Depp (as Thompson; who was in fact a friend of his) and Benicio del Toro (as Thompson's equally drug-indulging attorney) and directed by Terry Gilliam.

Thompson became best known for his book *Hell's Angels: The Strange and Terrible Saga of the Outlaw Motorcycle Gangs* (1967), based on a year he spent riding, drinking, and doing drugs with the bicker gang, while recording their lifestyle and life narratives (and ending with the gang rejecting him and beating him up). His approach to journalism, which he termed "Gonzo," was a highly personalized form of over-engaged renegade ethnography in which the reporter becomes such an active participant in the scene being covered that the reporter emerges as key figure in the final narrative. In keeping with the unconventionality of his life, at his death Thompson's ashes were shot from a cannon to the tune of Bob Dylan's "Mr. Tambourine Man."

Thompson came to be best known for some of his unconventional statements (2012), such as:

- I hate to advocate drugs, alcohol, violence, or insanity to anyone, but they've always worked for me. (Also expressed as: I wouldn't recommend sex, drugs or insanity for everyone, but they've always worked for me.)
- If you're going to be crazy, you have to get paid for it or else you're going to be locked up.
- You can turn your back on a person, but never turn your back on a drug, especially when it's waving a razor sharp hunting knife in your eye.
- The trouble with Nixon is that he's a serious politics junkie. He's totally hooked and like any other junkie, he's a bummer to have around, especially as President.

Thompson died of a self-inflicted gunshot wound in 2005. Of note, Thompson served as the model for the gun-toting, drug-using Uncle Duke character featured in Garry Trudeau's Doonesbury comic strip.

A number of individuals known for other things have written autobiographical books about the way drugs came into their lives at certain point and the deep impact it made. Key texts include those by Malcolm X, Claude Brown, Piri Thomas, and Manuel Torres.

In the years before his conversion to Islam, and his subsequent rise as an articulate, charismatic, and militant African American leader, Malcolm X (1987) relays in his autobiography his early life as a drug user and dealer. His encounter with drugs began while working as a shoeshine boy at the Roseland State Ballroom in Boston. While his job at first seemed to be about shining shoes, he quickly realized that a hidden aspect of the work, selling alcohol and marihuana and serving as a go-between for African American pimps and white customers, was where the real money could be made. Eventually he moved to New York where he worked selling marihuana, which he rolled into cigarettes ("reefers") and marketed to musicians in Harlem. For a period of time he even went on the road carrying a jar of marihuana "sticks" for sale to jazzmen in various East Coast locales. This association between the performance arts and drug use helped to create, in some circles, a street image of the drug user as a glamorous role worthy of emulation. One result, was not only drugs but jazz itself came to be widely condemned and its producers demonized. Yet, during the era that Malcolm X worked the streets, he found that in every band, a least half of the musicians smoked marihuana (many would also become addicted to heroin).

> I kept turning over my profit, increasing my supplies, and I sold reefers like a wild man. I scarcely slept; I was everywhere musicians congregated. A roll of money was in my pocket. Every day, I cleared at least fifty or sixty dollars. In those days ... this was a fortune to a seventeen-year-old Negro. I felt, for the first time in my life, that great feeling of free! Suddenly, now, I was the peer of the other young hustlers I had admired. (Malcolm X 1987:99)

Before long, Malcolm X came to the attention of the police. Under increasingly intense police scrutiny, he abandoned his drug business to pursue other hustles. Despite knowing that the police were watching him he continued to smoke marihuana and, at the same time, developed a dependence on cocaine. Cocaine offered him a way of handling the emotional stress of participating in robberies and running guns. This outlaw lifestyle came crashing down, however, when he was arrested and incarcerated on burglary charges. It was during his time in prison that Malcolm X experienced a radical personal transformation that involved both his conversion to Islam and his rejection of drug use. Consequently, Malcolm X was never swallowed up by the post-war heroin-boom on the streets of New York City, although he fell victim nonetheless to racial tensions and their internecine offspring.

Author and lecturer Claude Brown, several years younger than Malcolm X, had by age 13 developed a powerful attraction to heroin because of its popularity among the older boys and girls in the New York neighborhood where he grew up. As he described in his successful autobiographical book *Manchild in the Promised Land* (1965), initially, these older youth taught him to use marihuana. When they moved on to heroin, which, among other names was called "horse" at that time, he fervently wanted to join them. For several months during 1950 he was all but consumed by his craving for heroin:

> Horse was a new thing, not only in our neighborhood but in Brooklyn, the Bronx, and everyplace I went, uptown and downtown. It was like horse had just taken over. Everybody was talking about it. All the hip people were using it and snorting it and getting this new high.... I had been smoking reefers and had gotten high a lot of times, but I had the feeling that this horse was out of this world (Brown 1965:110-111).

Ultimately, Brown got his chance to try the drug.

> I couldn't believe it was really happening. I almost wanted to break out and laugh for joy, but I held back, and I snorted.... Something hit me right in the top of the head. It felt like a little spray of pepper on my brain.... Everything was getting rosy, beautiful. The sun got brighter in the sky and the whole day lit up and was twice as bright as it was before.... Everything was so slo-o-ow (Brown 1965:110{{en dahs}}111).

While some heroin users we have interviewed over the years have reported to us that their first exposure to the drug was extremely pleasurable, like love at first sight, leading them to adopt a long-term chase intended to relive the initial experience, Brown had a different reaction. After a few moments of euphoria:

My head seemed to stretch, and I thought my brain was going to burst. It was like a headache taking place all over the head at once and trying to break its way out. And then it seemed to get hot and hot and hot. And I was so slow.... I got scared. I'd never felt this way before in my life.... My guts felt like they were going to come out. Everything was bursting out all at once, and there was nothing I could do.... And I said, "O Lawd, if you'll just give me one more chance, one more chance, I'll never get high again" (Brown 1965:111).

Although he recovered from the terrors of his first high, he did not keep his vow. But he came in time to see the harsh toll drugs were taking on his friends and on his community and, with the support of a psychologist name Ernest Papanek of the Wiltwyck School for Boys, he vowed (and successfully was able) to redirect his life through education.

During the years early years in the lives of Malcolm X and Claude Brown, over in Spanish Harlem, Piri Thomas, a boy of mixed Puerto Rican and African American heritage, was a member of the younger post-war generation that was coming of age and coming into contact with drugs. He recalled one of his earliest encounters with marihuana at age 13. Drinking whiskey with several friends, one of them produced a "stick" of marihuana and asked if he would like to try it.

I felt its size. It was king-sized, a bomber. I put it to my lips and began to hiss my reserve away. It was going, going, going. I was gonna get a gone high. I inhaled. I held my nose, stopped up my mouth. I was gonna get a gone high ... a gone high ... a gone high ... and then the stick was gone, burnt to a little bit of a roach (Thomas 1967:58).

Like Malcolm X and Claude Brown, within a few years Thomas was using and selling marihuana and was soon addicted to heroin. Also like Malcolm X, he wound up in prison, where his habit switched to benzedrine, phenobarbital, alcohol, strained shellac, and whatever mind-altering drug the inmates could get their hands on that could take them away from the harsh realities of prison life. Ultimately, Piri too overcame his addiction and became an author, producing a memoir entitled *Down These Mean Streets*; additionally, he was very active in drug rehabilitation programs. Like Malcolm X's autobiography, Piri's book provides an engaging account of cruel racial prejudice, active discrimination, struggles to build a healthy identity in an oppressive drug-filled social environment, drug-shaped life experiences, and redemption following imprisonment.

Another autobiographic work of note focuses on the life history of Manuel Torres. In most ways, Torres' life story parallels those presented above. A gang member from his early teens during the 1950s, he tried heroin under circumstances not very different from those of Claude Brown, and like Brown his first experience with the drug was quite unpleasant. But his addict role model was his uncle and he encouraged Torres to try heroin a second time.

So I snort again and hey, it's like the shit really hit the fan.... you can't describe it. All the colors of Times Square tumble right over your forehead and explode in your eyeballs like a million, jillion shooting stars.... Everything's beautiful, and it's like nothing's happening baby but clear, crisp light (Rettig et al.: 33–34).

Soon Torres was snorting heroin on a daily basis. Then his uncle showed him how to skinpop (i.e., subcutaneous drug injection). Before long, Torres was injecting heroin four times a day, not to achieve a rush, but "just to maintain" a normal stability (Rettig et al. 1977:33). Indeed, this is a common motive for continuing to use addictive drugs that we have heard from many drug users. While they may enjoy some initial rush, as a long-term addict what they are mainly seeking is a return to normalcy, which for them has become drug-dependent. In the case of Torres, he began to "boost" (shoplift) to support his drug habit and then, like Malcolm X, turned to armed robbery, which led to arrest and imprisonment. Many years later, in reflecting on his life in his co-authored book *Manny, A Criminal Addict's Story*, Torres emphasized the political-economic origin of involvement with drugs among inner city youth. Responding to a statement about Durkheim's theory that the social role of criminals is to set the boundaries of acceptable behavior for the rest of society, Torres stated:

That's fine if you're on the right side of the tracks. But what if you are locked into the streets and locked out of the jobs because of your background or your dope habit? Hell, man, its simple for me to see, because I've been there. The social order created the drug problem and anything that comes of heroin addiction is their fault. Personal breakdowns are an aspect of social breakdowns (Rettig et al. 1977:175).

These four autobiographical accounts by Malcolm X, Claude Brown, Piri Thomas, and Manuel Torres, and related material (e.g., Pepper and Pepper 1984) poignantly reveal the development of the post-war urban drug scene.

Building on the image of the "cool" marihuana user of the depression and war years, the close of the Second World War ushered in a period of significant increase in heroin use and heroin addiction. This was sparked by the return of soldiers from parts of the world where drugs like heroin were readily available, and there was an opening up of the shipping lanes for the flow of drugs smuggled in by organized crime groups. The street addict, a social role in modern urban life (Stephens 1991), became a common sight on inner city streets, as each succeeding generation of youth, boys and girls alike, sought to prove themselves to their older peers by adopting the coveted persona of the hard-partying fearless drug adventurer. Other options and role models were few for youth who grew up in the times and places of these authors, and none offered, in their respective views, as much opportunity to prove their worth or face rejection in the one arena—the streets—that possessed any attainable potential of self-validation. In the wake of the heroin "plague," and other transformations Harlem and other US inner cities changed dramatically. These were the years that ghettos were being reconfigured as hyperghettos and life changed dramatically for residents of the abandoned cores of the metropolis (Singer et al. 2006; Wacquant 2001).

As a result of the myriad technoeconomic changes that began to emerge during the 1960s, ethnic-minority working-class labor became increasingly expendable, as seen in the steeply rising level of poverty in the inner city in subsequent years. Critical to this change, the sense of community, which was revived after the migration of African Americans from the South and Puerto Ricans from the Island to inner cities, and even survived grinding poverty and the fierce racial discrimination that undercut self-esteem and self-worth encountered in northern and mid-western metropolises, was shattered by widespread drug addiction among individuals who had nowhere to turn for drug money except robbery, burglary, prostitution, and other crimes against themselves, their families, and their neighbors.

Drugs, for many, however, led to arrest and imprisonment as the War on Drugs became a multimillion-dollar industry and drug policies became an increasingly powerful institutionalization of racial segregation. The result was the creation of a social space comprising the ghetto and the prison united by a revolving door, with drugs available in both sectors. From the outside, this structure could be imagined as a thing unto itself produced and maintained by weak family values, lassitude, and immorality. Unseen, of course, in such condescending understandings were the underlying structures of economically driven racial discrimination that were the true drivers of the system. In this, the mechanics of the creation of useless categories of people, and their many less visible uses for the larger society, came to full fruition.

Not all introductions to psychotropic drugs were as dramatic as those just described. In her autobiography (1911), entitled *Twenty Years at Hull-House,* noted social reformer Jane Addams confessed an episode of drug use during her teen years. In this encounter with opium, she and a group of friends at a female seminary were inspired by their reading of Thomas de Quincey's widely read book. Wrote Hull (1911:46):

> We solemnly consumed small white powders at intervals during an entire long holiday, but no mental reorientation took place, and the suspense and excitement did not even permit us to grow sleepy. About four o'clock on the weird afternoon, the young teacher whom we had been obliged to take into our confidence grew alarmed over the whole performance, took away our de Quincey and all the remaining powders, administered an emetic to each of the five aspirants for sympathetic understanding of all human experience, and sent us to our separate rooms with a stern command to appear at family worship after supper "whether we were able to or not."

As this example suggests, at a time when opium was a legal drug, de Quincey's literary influence was significant, inspiring brief attempts at drug experimentation in various individuals who gained recognition for their work in and out of literary circles. Their writings, in turn, helped to maintain a level of social interest in the drug experience among readers.

DRUGS IN SOCIETY

It is fair to designate a whole genre of literature as "depictions of the impact of drugs on society," namely writings that in whole or in part can be read as fictionalized accounts of the ways drugs have shaped human social life in a particular time and place. Exemplary is the novella *The Crying of Lot 49* (1966), seen by some as one of the best literary works of the 20th century, by Thomas Pynchon. Living up to Pynchon's reputation for constructing labyrinthine plots crammed with innumerable interlinked riddles and cultural references, the novella tells the convoluted tale of a woman named Oedipa Maas involved in investigating the encrypted evidence of a mysterious conflict between two private mail distribution companies and of a suite of exotic characters she encounters during her inquiry. Included in this voyage into the netherworld of human imagination in an extensively fragmented and chaotic society is Maas's encounter with a group called Inamorati Anonymous, which is dedicated to helping people avoid falling in love, which is said to be the worst addiction of all.

Despite this assertion, the novella provides an account of the heavy toll drugs and drug culture have taken on the quality of human communication and the depth of human relationship. While drug use takes place throughout the book, its impact on two of the characters is of note. The first is Mucho, Oedipa's husband, whose life is derailed by LSD, as he loses his identity and sense of self as a result of the drug's effects. But he does not see it that way at first. Defending LSD, Mucho explains his reason for taking LSD in these terms:

> You take it because it's good. Because you hear and see things, even smell them, taste like you never could. Because the world is so abundant. No end to it, baby. You're an antenna, sending your pattern out across a million lives a night, and they're your lives too (Pynchon :1965:118).

Similarly, Dr. Hilarius, Oedipa's psychologist loses his capacity to even listen to Oedipa as he experiments with LSD, mescaline, psilocybin, and other drugs as a therapeutic tools. In due course, drug use drives Dr. Hilarius crazy.

One reading of this book is certainly that drug use (or at least 1960s drug culture) contributed to an ever-more fragmented and divided society in which each lonely individual must cope both with a suffocating sense of endless isolation and with confusion about the borderline between reality and illusion. Pynchon's view of drugs, in short, was not a pretty picture: behind the claims of those like Huxley or Burroughs about the power of drugs to open the mind and free the self from the straitjacket of social convention, Pynchon saw chaos, seclusion, and social disintegration.

The book *Crank* (2003) is semi-autobiographical verse novel by Ellen Hopkins. In the book, targeted like many fictional works with a strong anti-drug message to junior high and high school readers, Hopkins shares the stormy and often troublesome relationship between Kristina, a character that is based on her own daughter, and what is referred to as the "monster," crystal methamphetamine. Kristina is introduced to the monster when separated from her controlling mother and visits her deadbeat and drug-involved father in another town. Under the influence of the drug, her personality (and name) is transformed as she becomes the fast-paced, risk-taking, Bree. Left behind is the sweet, gifted, and conventional Kristina persona. Under the spell of meth, Kristina/Bree's grades plunge, her relationships with family and friends are disrupted, and her involvement with drug-using boys accelerates. Ultimately she hits bottom when she is raped by a drug dealer and becomes pregnant. While she keeps the baby, and this lowers her level of drug use, her meth consumption continues to the end of the book. While a certain amount of space is opened for alternative interpretations by the pregnancy, it is evident that a message of the book is that drugs destroy lives and relationships, and that humans are at risk of this ever-lurking monster.

The title of *Diary of a Drug Fiend* (1922), by wealthy English author, occultist, poet, communalist, magician and admitted anti-semite Aleister Crowley, leaves little doubt about the centrality of drugs to the book. Believed to be based on Crowley own experimental use of drugs (which he meticulously documented) and eventual drug addiction, the book chronicles the lives of the characters Peter Pendragon and Louise Laleham, on a heroin and cocaine binge and drug-craving journey across Europe. While their exploration of drug use begins in a light-hearted way, ultimately, on the verge of committing suicide, they are saved from the maniacal evil of drugs by a magician (as was Crowley for a time) who shows them, via a visit to the occult retreat known as the Abbey of Thelema (a Crowley mainstay), how to impose their will over self-destructive urges. The book offers a graphic description of the absolute horrors of drug addiction and treachery of hitting bottom, but seems also to suggest that drugs can be wonderful tools if managed appropriately.

DENS OF INIQUITY

While various drug use settings are described in literary sources, few have attracted as much appeal as the so-called opium den, the very label for which conjures up a mix of scandalous erotic and psychotropic experience (made manifest by the fact that lights were low and beds were a common furnishing) that often transcends socially reinforced ethnic boundaries. Historically, opium dens have been darkly associated with the Chinese, overlooking the fact that it was the British who forced their colonial opium harvest from India onto China and helped to create a widespread drug problem there. The British armed forces killed Chinese in two wars (the so-called Boxer Rebellions) to insure the profits of a vast drug market in China, only to have the Chinese be blamed as the pushers who lured the innocent (read: white women) into their shadowy lairs of drug abandonment. In this cultural sleight-of-hand is revealed the social mechanics of the making of the useless other, and why this other is usefully made.

Opium dens appear in various well-known literary products. In the Sherlock Holmes story, first published in 1891, "The Man with the Twisted Lip" by Sir Arthur Conan Doyle, for example, Dr. Watson, Holmes's collaborator and alter ego, searches an opium den in the East End of London to find Isa Whitney, the husband of one of his wife's friends. In the den, Watson discovers Holmes, disguised as an old man, seeking information on a new case he has taken on. At the time, sale and use of opium were legal in England, although this would change within a few years.

In the 1884 short story, "The Gate of a Hundred Sorrows," Rudyard Kipling in his first published work (written when he was 18 years old) tells the history of a Chinese opium den in India. The language of the story bespeaks the attitudes of the day. Writes Kipling through his narrator, a customer of the Gate of a Hundred Sorrow:

> I used to go there, and, somehow, I have never got away from it since. Mind you, though, the Gate was a respectable place in Fung-Tching's time where you could be comfortable, and not at all like the chandoo-khanas where the niggers go. No; it was clean and quiet, and not crowded. Of course, there were others beside us ten and the man; but we always had a mat apiece with a wadded woollen head-piece, all covered with black and red dragons and things; just like a coffin in the corner.

In Charles Dickens's final (and uncompleted) novel, *The Mystery of Edwin Drood,* a graphic account is provided of an London East End opium den and its customers. A friend of Dickens, J. T. Field recorded that Dickens was quite aware of such places and that he had accompanied the famous author in the summer of 1869 on visits to some lock-up houses, watch-houses, and opium dens (with a police escort) (Kitton 1897).

The story begins as choirmaster John Jasper, a man who is secretly in love with his vocal student Rosa Bud, the fiancée of his nephew, Edwin Drood, is leaving an opium den. Sometime later he visits the den again, but when he leaves at dawn the operator of the den, a haggard woman known as the Princess Puffer, comes running after him and follows him to his home. This action apparently stems from something John Jasper told her while under the stuporous effects of opium. As noted, the novel was never finished so the substance of Jasper's drug-induced revelation is not revealed. But there is clear indication that the opium den, while legal at the time, was viewed by the higher social classes as a dark and threatening place entangled with all manner of socially disapproved behaviors. Notably, Dickens' death, which caused the book to be unfinished, followed a period of poor health and his use of laudanum to both help him sleep and cope with the pain he felt in his legs.

To express indulgence in life's most exotic pleasures, his novel *The Picture of Dorian Gray*, first published in the final decade of the 19th century, Oscar Wilde (1890) has his character Dorian visit various opium dens of London. Gray, aware and deeply worried that someday his youthful beauty will fade, is willing to sell his soul to retain an impressive image of himself captured in portrait by an artist friend. Wilde's incorporation of opium dens, located in remote and dilapidated spaces of the city, have been interpreted by critics as representing the disreputable areas of Gray's personality. Expressing Wilde's own contempt of Victorian morality, Dorian seeks out these dens of the underworld after committing a murder and hopes in them to forget the horror of his actions by losing consciousness in a drug-induced torpor. Although he has a container of opium in his home, Dorian leaves the safety of his comfortable social environment to journey to the murky dens that reflect the deepening degradation of his soul, as drugs come to reflect in the story a degradation of the human spirit.

In *Delta of Venus Erotica* (1977) by Anaïs Nin, there is a short story in which the lead character finds herself in an opium den. Nin was a French-Cuban author, who lived in France and later in Cuba and the United States. Over the course of her life, Nin had romantic relationships with many leading male literary figures, including Henry Miller, John Steinbeck, Gore Vidal, James Agee, and Lawrence Durrell. As part of a voyage of self-discovery as a woman, she wrote journals, novels, critical studies, essays, short stories, as well as erotica, and these earned her international acclaim. Stories in *Delta of Venus Erotica* dealt with many taboo subjects including abuse, incest, homosexuality, prostitution, infidelity, and pedophilia. In the story in question, the female lead character Elena enters what appears to be a smoke-filled mosque. Nin writes (1977:134),

> It was a huge room surrounded by a gallery of alcoves furnished only with mats and little lamps. Everyone was wearing kimonos. Elena was handed one. And then she understood. This was an opium den; the lights veiled; people lying down, indifferent to the newcomers; a great peace; no sustained conversations, but a sign now and then. A few for whom opium awakened desire lay in the darkest corners, spoon-fashion, as if asleep.

The increasingly erotic description proceeds, leaving an image of the opium den as a site of drug-awakening sexuality. Notably in another story, *Children of the Albatross"* (2004:153), Nin wrote "In the world of the dreamer there was solitude: all the exaltations and joys came in the moment of preparation for living. They took place in solitude. But with action came anxiety, and the sense of insuperable effort made to match the dream, and with it came weariness, discouragement, and the flight into solitude again. And then in solitude, in the opium den of remembrance, the possibility of pleasure again." While taking the visitor to the edge of proper society, drug dens in Nin's hand are associated more with pleasure than pain, affirming the existence of alternative drug themes in literature.

In "The Lost Mine," a short story by murder mystery writer Agatha Christie, her well-known dapper detective character, Hercule Poirot, is forced against his will to conduct part of his investigation in London in a Limehouse opium den "right in the heart of Chinatown" (Christie 1924:221). This establishment is described as being of "the lowest description" (Christie 1924:221), asserting a rather different view of the opium den than that presented by Nin. In effect, this contrast of Nin and Christie, in terms of their respective places within society and the degree of conventionality with which they approached their use of the opium den setting within their writing, says much about the contrastive messages about drug users, drugs, and drug use environments found in literature, as discussed more fully below.

DRUGS, LITERATURE, AND THE ISSUE OF USEFULNESS

As this review suggests, some writers (at certain times in their lives or their whole lives) hold the view that drugs and the altered consciousness they produce are a kind of psychological fuel that opens their minds to new levels of unconventional understanding and broadens their vision as an author, or, at least, are needed almost medicinally to manage various physical and emotional symptoms enabling them to be physically able to write. Certainly, many of the authors we have discussed lived lives badly damaged by drugs, and they often describe their suffering (and that of those around them) in their books and other works, directly or indirectly. As a result, one can find harsh images of drug use and drug users in literature, but contrary images are also abundant and there are those writers who firmly defend drug use as a vital component of their literary quest. One can look at the life of the writer or at what the writer has produced in his/her lifetime and find quite varied messages about drugs. This is not surprising because there are those writers who define their life work as transcending conventionality and the barriers to life experience and understanding imposed by society, and there are other writers who are inspired by quite different visions of the purposes of transmitting thoughts, feelings, plot lines, character descriptions, and story narratives into formats that can be read by others (e.g., providing enjoyment). Some writers, quite literally, write against society and are therefore less likely to demonize those on the edges of the social order than they are the elites who rule from the powerful center. Writers who feel somewhat outside of society or even in conflict with it, may, if they make use of the drug user in their work, be somewhat more humanizing in their portrayal or at least more tolerant or less condemning. Othering of the drug user, however, is still common enough in literature, as exploring the edges of social life is a reliable means of affirming orthodox values. In sum, while the drug user as boogey man theme can be found in literature, it is far from the only theme to be found there, and hence the take-home messages for readers will differ depending on what they read and who they read and what they know of the impact of drugs on writers' own lives.

Whatever their stance towards drugs, given the extensive and for some quite heavy use of drugs among the creators of literature, writers as a group can be said to contradict prevailing stereotypes about drug users. Some of the most admired and celebrated works of literature were produced by drug users and possibly while they were under the influence of drugs. Many writers with solid reputations as accomplished producers of fiction, poetry, journalistic accounts, and related matter have entertained and educated despite (or, at times because of) their drug use. Yet, somewhat magically, their creations are separated from their lives and their lives are separated from those of less socially accomplished drug users, especially minority and street drug users, a type of fictional creation of social reality worthy of any the authors reviewed in this chapter.

CHAPTER FIVE

Picture This

Pictorial Construction of Drug Users
in the World of Film

I n the process of Othering addicts, there is hardly a more effective medium than pictorial representations. The relatively brief historical span
of the concept of addiction as a feature of public discourse began to yield
drawings (such as Hogarth's etchings) in the 18th century, with additional
depictions by cartoonists such as Nast in the 19th and early 20th centuries.
The introduction of photography and motion pictures, however, opened
myriad possibilities for conceiving and making pictorial narratives about the
nature and process of addiction. This chapter focuses on the development
of moving pictures, in part because even the earliest filmmakers showed
special interest in drug users and the effects of drugs. Films, and later videos
extended the powers of representation far beyond those of drawings or still
photographs, giving latitude for extended narratives about the development
of addiction and its maintenance and treatment. Films have about two hours
to extend the narrative, and television series such as *The Wire* and *Breaking
Bad* have taken these potentials into previously uncharted dramatic territory
in terms of character development and time depth of the addictive process.
In this examination of the history of motion pictures on addiction, we use
anthropological findings from drug-user research in our analyses. In our categorization of film portrayals of drug use, we identify a set of common themes
about this behavior frequently communicated through this medium. We
avoid discussion of the considerable inventory of psychedelic and so-called
"stoner" films because they do not typically deal with the issue of addiction.

DRAWINGS AND PHOTOS

In 1874, when *Harper's Weekly* wanted to tell its readers about the depths of
depravity caused by drunkenness, the magazine relied on illustrators, including the famous Thomas Nast, to portray the dangers of drink using images

The Social Value of Drug Addicts: The Uses of the Useless, by Merrill Singer and J. Bryan Page, 121–152.

of stupefied women, careless men, and desperate, abandoned children who either directly or indirectly suffered from the effects of drunkenness. These depictions helped to fuel the growing sentiment against alcohol consumption that eventually led to the enactment of prohibition. The power of visual images, even ones drawn from the imagination of the illustrator, to move a mass readership's perceptions was at that time just in the early process of development. The introduction of photography, which was capable of capturing images of real behaviors as they occurred, and to claim (if somewhat questionably so) the netting of objective real-time reality, made it possible for a profusion of images to appear in printed media. Photography brought to the attention of large readerships the conditions and state of the clientele in saloons and bars. If the WCTU or another temperance group created a disturbance in front of a bar, photographers could capture that moment and transmit it to people who were not present via newspapers or magazines. Carry Nation and her hatchet became media icons as a result of her frequent appearances in front of news cameras.

With regard to other drugs, photographs of users and drug clinics received print media attention as objects of public concern. For example, *Modern Medicine* featured pictures of activity outside a drug clinic in 1920, and *The Literary Digest* published a photo of narcotics officers inspecting a haul of confiscated drugs in 1923 (Morgan 1981:113,114,119). These presentations, however, were essentially journalistic activities aimed at making the reading public aware of happenings in their communities or in the rest of the country.

Although the news media, in their use of still photography and editorial cartoons, came to exert considerable influence over how the public perceived drug use and drug users, as well as the people who opposed them, the introduction and elaboration of moving pictures provided an especially rich opportunity for presenting compelling narratives about these topics, not just with documentary reports but with dramatizations of personal experience. Film brings especially powerful images into public consciousness. Analysts and media specialists constantly work to define the power of images produced in ever-greater profusion by the photographic and digital devices that give access to all phases of the human condition. This much is known: it takes less than one second for an image to be recognized by a human viewer. Gladwell's (2005) interpretation of this phenomenon suggests that volumes of knowledge, emotion, and experience can be evoked by a single image. In a medium that has images moving and shifting across the human visual field, the possibilities for evocation are endless. With this principle in mind, we review and examine content, quality, and intent of visual media with considerably more focus on film and video than on still pictures. Our review concentrates on the portrayal of the addict and the cultural context of addiction in pictorial media, in other words in the cultural construction of the addict within the film industry

A thorough inventory of both documentary and entertainment films, especially taking into account films produced outside of the United States and Western Europe, makes a comprehensive critical treatment of drugs in film impossible except in a multi-volume format. In a single chapter, we can only hope to point out some of the influential films that focus on the nature and impact of addiction, as that concept has been constructed in Western discourse. Therefore, we only attempt to offer a perspective on how films have portrayed drug users' experiences, with special attention to the impact of addiction. We also mostly avoid the exploitation films (films produced with the intent of attracting an audience that seeks titillation) unless they have the trappings of educational cautionary tales, such as the infamous *Reefer Madness*. Most of the movies reviewed here could be construed as "mainstream," intended to attract a general audience. In our review, we point out homologies that contribute to the audience's conceptualization of addiction, as well as unique features that add innovative perspectives on addiction.

HOW TO CONSTRUCT A DRUG-USING OTHER

Films present "an irresistible opportunity to feed the audience's appetite for spectacle, for something out of the ordinary—in short, for Otherness" (Donally 2012:1). Some very early films focused on drug use as it was known before the turn of the 20th century, including titles such as *Chinese Opium Den* (1895), a kinetoscope film only 30 seconds long (Starks 1982:13). Films like this tended to focus on exoticism, with exoticized portrayals of Chinese opium dens, white slavery, and even the infamous Fu Manchu. In that sense, they could be termed exploitation films, although that variety of film did not emerge for another decade or so. The true motivation for making films about opium users may be related to the notion that they were known to have fantastic dreams when intoxicated with that drug, and early filmmakers were eager to render special effects that gave the audience the feeling of having an opium dream. *Rube in an Opium Joint* (1905) depicted this kind of experience, as did *Rêves d'un Fumeur d'Opium (Dreams of an Opium Smoker)* (1906), a very early French film (Starks 1982:13). A Danish filmmaker and actor, Holger-Madsen released *Opiumsdrömmen* (1914) depicting very explicit opium dreams. Stuart Kinder, a British director, put out *The Opium Cigarettes*

(1914) which included "weird visions," and the famous German director, Robert Reinert, who produced *Opium* (1919), included dream sequences (Starks 1982:15). Given the abundance of subject matter for a new medium, the pioneering directors' decisions to include movies about opium smoking in their portfolios testifies to the specific attractiveness of this kind of content during the early days of filmmaking. The Victorian cultural context in which these films found an audience that included large numbers of people who were deeply confused about sexuality. In this kind of cultural environment, titillation often involved views of very foreign behaviors, practiced by phenotypically distinctive people. Opium's identification with the "mysterious Orient" and its known addictive properties layered implications of behavior outside the bounds of propriety, even sexual enslavement, into the audience appeal of these early films.

By the 1930s, with the addition of sound tracks to the motion pictures, all of the tools were in place to construct well-acted, compellingly written dramas about the ecstasy and misery of drug use for audiences that might not like being close to drug users in person but could be entertained by their alleged behaviors in darkened theaters and at some distance. The same ingredients could also be combined into laughable attempts at disinformation and spurious propaganda.

Portrayals of drug users in film give the beholder a sense of the users' humanity, fallibility, and culpability. Whether the protagonists are high-functioning upper-middle-class alcoholics, as in *Leaving Las Vegas, The Lost Weekend, Night into Morning, Days of Wine and Roses,* and *Come Fill the Cup,* or crumbling street-based addicts, as in *The Panic in Needle Park, Trainspotting,* and *Christianne F.,* the best of the films about addiction convey those protagonists' merits, flaws, and impairment thanks to highly intelligent and astute script writing and often superb acting. The film medium gives abundant opportunities to impart nuance and idiosyncrasy to a character's personal profile, yet in aggregate, the homologies among on-screen addict characters are so strong that adverse stereotypic configurations emerge. These homologies include accounts of how the addictive process begins, description of deteriorating social relations, desperate behavior involving money, involvement in frantic crimes and misdemeanors, body-wrenching withdrawal pangs, recidivism, betrayal of intimate others, prostitution, and eventually, either long-term and difficult withdrawal, continued addiction and all of its accompanying sufferings, or death.

Whether the films are of high or low quality, the homologies listed above obtain across the several sub-genres that have arisen since the dawn of the moving-picture era. The first film generally recognized as part of the addiction film genre was *Human Wreckage,* which was released in 1923, and unfortunately is now believed to be a lost film (Starks 1982:48). It belongs to the sub-genre that we call "biographical cautionary tales." Both memoire-derived and fictional narratives belong to this genre, which also includes such films as *Reefer Madness, Monkey on My Back, Ray, The Basketball Diaries, Marijuana—Assassin of Youth,* and *Lady Sings the Blues.* Each gives an account of how a protagonist begins to use a drug, seeks alternative social relations, becomes desperate for money to obtain more of their drug of choice (or as it is portrayed, drug of domination), commits crimes, agonizes through a bout of torturous withdrawal pangs, relapses, and compromises personal values and dignity in pursuit of drugs. Presentations of *Human Wreckage,* for example often were accompanied by a lecture given by the protagonist's widow, Mrs. Wallace Reid. According to her lectures, her husband was attempting to recover from "the fast life" shared by Hollywood stars, having checked into a sanitarium, when he died suddenly of complications related to withdrawal from morphine. Reid's death elicited sympathy, but it also represented an opportunity for Hollywood to cash in on that sympathy. The film's very title embodies the societal construction of the damaged and worthless drug user.

At least one of the films mentioned above misrepresents practically all of the components of the sub-genre—*Reefer Madness,* because it is purely a fabrication based on the most lurid journalistic accounts of aberrant behavior connected with young white people who smoked an evil drug: marihuana. Its narrative excesses are legendary, and have been fodder for great hilarity among young audiences from 1970 to the present. Nevertheless, the fact that the same components that appear in far more meritorious films also appear in *Reefer Madness* raises the question of how these components became fixed as part of a narrative about a drug that only rarely involves addiction. Likely sources include the first book-length addiction narrative in English literature—de Quincey's *Diary of an English Opium Eater* (1822) (discussed in Chapter 4) and some of the 18th and 19th century tracts and books about heavy drinking and alcoholism (discussed in Chapter 3). Given that kind of material, with all the familiar elements of process from initial casual use to escalating self-destruction to eventual withdrawal or death, it is easy to imagine the screenplay writer of *Reefer Madness,* Paul Franklin, referring to the works of Thomas de Quincey; Joseph Livesey, the great English temperance advocate; or American temperance author Timothy Shay Arthur in formulating the addiction narrative he wished to insert into his film. All of these writings contained the key elements of initial social use, escalation, loss of social support, and undesirable outcomes. Once Franklin had conceived of the framework of addictive career, it was easy to contrive situations in which the actors could clutch their throats and growl, "I gotta have more reefer!" To our knowledge, no one who has spent time in the company of marihuana smokers, even the heaviest smokers, has ever heard such an utterance except when watching *Reefer Madness*. Acts of violence, attempted rape, and gibbering madness are some of the other fabrications that Franklin slathered into his screenplay.

Franklin's phony contrivances notwithstanding, some grains of truth could be derived from his oeuvre. For example, his Jimmy character drives recklessly under the influence of marihuana and runs over a pedestrian. Most of the research that has tested acute effects of Cannabis on drivers of automobiles has found that psychomotor function and acuity were reduced and reaction time increased under the influence (e.g., Sewell et al. 2009). The high frequency of detecting alkaloids of Cannabis in the blood of auto-accident fatalities testifies further to the veracity of this particular aspect of the effects of Cannabis (Grotenhermen et al. 2007). Also, although the film grotesquely exaggerated the laughter associated with cannabis use, it remains true that laughter is one of the drug's most commonly reported effects, even cross-culturally (e.g., Page et al. 1980:125). We can find evidence of how abject Franklin's ignorance of marihuana's acute effects in the fact that he failed to include in his narrative the hunger cravings referred by users as the "munchies," an effect that is widely reported among users in the United States and elsewhere (cf. Dreher 1982; Rubin and Comitas 1975; Page and Carter 1980).

Reefer Madness did, however, go out of its way to exaggerate the things that the newly recruited marihuana smokers were willing to do under the drug's influence. Spontaneous, inexplicable violence, overwhelming lust, and general loss of impulse control all played parts in depicting how marihuana could ruin the lives of innocent white youth. Again, having spent considerable time observing male Costa Rican cannabis users in various contexts, and at dosages far higher than any possible in the United States in the 1930s (cf. Page 1983; Page and Carter 1980; Page et al. 1988), Page saw no evidence of the kinds of behavioral aberrations depicted in *Reefer Madness*. Much earlier than Page's observational experience, Becker (1953) reported on the process observed in Chicago of learning the relatively subtle effects of cannabis and how to appreciate them. Far from causing naïve users to launch into debauchery, Becker's account of the process of learning to use marihuana required the guidance of experienced "veterans" to point out the nature of the drug's effects and how to recognize them. None of this process received any attention in *Reefer Madness,* except techniques for smoking marihuana cigarettes.

Reefer Madness's attempt to construct a fraudulent Otherness in its marihuana-smoking characters also has a certain poignancy, because the film narrative eventually directs some level of pity at the naïve victims of the scourge that is cannabis. Rather than fully demonizing the youths (who are white and middle class) who tried marihuana for "kicks," the film either executes them or discards them as felons or mental patients with little hope of redemption. The narrator expresses the hope that people who see this film will "tell your children" in an effort to keep these kinds of outcomes from continuing.

Perhaps because *Reefer Madness* was an early attempt to exert influence on the public perception of a drug's consumers, it feels especially contrived and false. Its makers relied heavily on their audience's lack of any direct knowledge about the drug and its effects. By the early 1970s when *Reefer Madness* was re-discovered and re-released, millions of people in the United States had at least tried marihuana, and their familiarity with the drug and its effects converted the film from cautionary drama to uproarious comedy without having to change anything. In 1992, a stage production/take-off of *Reefer Madness* played for a year in Chicago, and in 1998 a stage musical version opened in Los Angeles, eventually finding its way to the off-Broadway scene in 2001, but closing after a few performances. Showtime's 2005 movie version of *Reefer Madness* incorporated the musical numbers of the stage show, adhering to the original movie's plot until the last third, when it devolved into a zombie apocalypse, either commenting on the perception that marihuana smokers become zombie-like[1] or seeking to exploit the growing interest in and domestication of monsters and other worldly beings in 21st century books, films and TV programming.

Another movie, written by Hildegarde Stadie and entitled simply *Marihuana* was released in 1936 by the same person who distributed *Reefer Madness,* Dwain Esper, Stadie's husband. It followed the same exploitative and disinformative path, linking marihuana smoking with forbidden sex, gratuitous violence, and illicit activity, and finally adding a new wrinkle—an early expression of the "steppingstone theory." The film's protagonist, having embarked on the road to perdition, progresses to the point of injecting heroin. According to that theory, shortly after a young person tries marihuana, the weed smoker rapidly becomes the heroin injector. Otherwise, Stadie followed the formula laid out by Franklin, including the casual encounter, the recreational exposure, the undesirable behavior, and the slide into criminality.

Stadie also disposed of her characters and warned the audience to beware of this "new" drug menace to the cream of American (i.e., white, middle and upper class) youth.

Cocaine had received cinematic attention before the era of talkies, including silent versions of Sherlock Holmes mysteries released in the early 20th century, and notably *The Mystery of the Leaping Fish* (1916), a spoof on Sherlock Holmes starring Douglas Fairbanks Sr. as cocaine-injecting detective Coke Ennyday (Starks 1982:38). The film expresses a surprisingly light-hearted view of regular cocaine and opium use at a time when these drugs were being criminalized. During the mid-1930s, *The Pace That Kills,* (also entitled *The Cocaine Fiends*) used a plot line that rapidly plunged the protagonist into full-bore criminality in a matter of minutes. Cocaine's intrinsic seductiveness became the centerpiece in the principal characters' fall into sin and perdition. This relatively short (just under one hour), badly edited film also introduced a sub-plot that would become a major theme in other films about addiction—young junkies in love. Two of the main characters, Fanny and Eddie, begin their relationship with the occasional use of cocaine (presented as "headache powders" to the naïve first-time users) that escalates rapidly into addiction, loss of employment, and eventually prostitution. One of the peculiarities of this particular film is the nomenclature used about the drugs, a confusion noted by Starks (1982:37) regarding the filmmakers' perceptions of opiate and cocaine effects. There are multiple examples. Cocaine is called "dope" by the underworld characters, but in our experience, users have never called it that. As Fanny and Eddie progress in their relationship, she invites him to a "snowbird party." This term may have been current to denote cocaine users, and at that point in the film, the two lovers were snorting powder cocaine. Nevertheless, although we have heard "snow" as a gloss for cocaine, users have never been called "snowbirds" in our experience. Later, in his addictive desperation, Eddie tells Fanny that he needs another "shot," but no injection paraphernalia are in evidence. He later acknowledges that he is a "hophead," a term usually employed in the early 20th century to denote opiate users. This mish-mosh of terms seems to indicate that the moviemakers were somewhat confused about the properties of the drug that was the ostensible focus of the film. Later, toward the end of the film, Eddie's sister finds him in what appears to be a Chinese opium den. In their zeal to titillate and exploit, Willis Kent (producer) and William A. O'Connor (director) carelessly mixed cocaine, nightclub life, opium smoking, and prostitution into a hodgepodge of not-very-believable drug-use practices. The opium den seems a particularly gratuitous exoticism for this particular plot line although it was consistent with the content of previous movies. Nevertheless, we now know enough about cocaine use to recognize that opioids can be helpful in mitigating the cocaine "crash," a process involving dopamine depletion that occurs after a long run of cocaine use. Cocaine users resort to alcohol, tranquilizers, or opioid drugs to ease the discomfort of the post-cocaine "crash." In showing Eddie in an opium den, even *The Cocaine Fiends* contains, if perhaps accidently so, a grain of truth.

The arrest of Robert Mitchum in September of 1948 provided an opportunity for a woman named Lila Leeds to exploit the circumstances through a film entitled *She Shoulda Said "No"!* She and Mitchum, who had been smoking marihuana since his youth, had been arrested for possessing and smoking marihuana, and although the charges were eventually overturned in 1951, the notoriety brought by the incident made it possible to produce a film exploiting marihuana's potential (still largely unknown by the US population) for harming American youth.

Films of the 1950s and early 1960s tended to avoid marihuana as a topic. Perhaps this avoidance represented the general conservatism of the times. For example, Prohibition had been over for 20 years, but the surviving temperance movement still had enough strength to stop electronic media's advertising of liquor in the 1950s (Pennock 2007:5). Even the otherwise gritty, inner-city drama *Blackboard Jungle* demurred in 1955 at mentioning marihuana, which undoubtedly was present in such settings. The presence of rock and roll constituted the major menace portrayed in that film. Among youth during this time, marihuana use was found disproportionately in inner city areas among minority youth, a group that had never been the concern of the earlier wave of over-the-top cinematic portrayals of this drug's consumption.

Heroin use, however, became a major topic in prominent films released in the 1950s and '60s, especially in the biographical genre. *The Man with the Golden Arm* (1955) was a film adaptation of a novel by Nelson Algren that had, unlike the exploitation films that preceded it, the multiple advantages of a skilled director (Otto Preminger, known for resisting efforts to sanitize portrayals of drug use in film), high production values, an Oscar-nominated musical score by Elmer Bernstein, and a first-rate cast, including Frank Sinatra in the lead role, and Arnold Stang, Robert Strauss, and Darren McGavin as supporting characters. Its critical reception was enthusiastic, netting Oscar nominations for Sinatra's performance, Bernstein's score, and art and set decoration in a black-and-white film.

The Man with the Golden Arm, however, ran afoul of the Motion Picture Association of America (MPAA) because that body concluded that the film's content was not acceptable to be shown to a public audience.[2] Because of its focus on heroin use, the MPAA found *The Man with the Golden Arm* to be unacceptable, despite the fact that films of such poor quality as *Reefer Madness* and *She Shoulda Said "No"!* had received code approval. Possibly, *The Man with the Golden Arm* presented too sympathetic a view of the addict or addiction for the MPAA's taste, although its torturous withdrawal scene, during which the protagonist (played by Sinatra, who had observed patients in drug treatment centers to prepare for the role) withdrew from heroin, amid convulsions, shakes, shivers, and apparent cramps, certainly did not make heroin use seem desirable. Eventually, the MPAA relented and granted the film a code, and box office and critical success ensued. This movie's single most arresting feature involved a sequence in which the protagonist had himself locked in a room in order to bear the rigors of "cold turkey" withdrawal alone. These scenes later became de rigueur for biographical movies that included heroin addiction, despite the fact that our own field work and that of our colleagues (Agar 1973; Page and Salazar 1997; Rosenbaum 1981) found withdrawal symptoms to be far less histrionic and more flu-like (which is not necessarily mild) than those portrayed in the biographical movies (and there is no doubt that the fear of going through withdrawal can help propel continued drug use).

Shortly after the release of *The Man with the Golden Arm, Monkey on My Back* (1957) became the first biographical film on addiction under MPAA's revised policy on formerly "taboo" content. This film about Barney Ross, a former boxer and war hero, and his struggles with morphine addiction, gave Cameron Mitchell ample opportunity to portray various desperate situations experienced by Ross during the course of his addiction. It also placed in the broad public lexicon a phrase (dating to the late 1800s, although not originally about drug use) that had come to denote the rigors of addiction for street based heroin users—"monkey on my back." This phrase, which historically referred to an evil or upsetting spirit, came to be widely used in drug scenes in the United States and elsewhere, finding its way into an Aerosmith song (about the recognition of band members of their need to overcome drug abuse), and even becoming an expression used by Spanish heroin users when they begin to feel the symptoms of withdrawal (Page and Salazar 1997).

Alcoholism was apparently somewhat less taboo than other forms of addiction, as *The Lost Weekend* (1945) demonstrated through its critical success and its lack of trouble with the MPAA. Ray Milland won an academy award for his portrayal of an alcoholic writer's struggles with alcohol addiction. The film also received awards for best picture, best director (Billy Wilder) and best screenplay. As with *The Man with the Golden Arm, The Lost Weekend* had significant cinematic advantages of talented direction, writing, and acting, and an innovative musical score, an early example of using the theremin (an electronic musical instrument played without touch) to achieve effects of disorientation and pathos. *The Lost Weekend* had a notable advantage over *The Man with the Golden Arm* and *Monkey on my Back* in that its protagonist was an upper-middle-class writer living in New York, rather than a struggling ex-convict or a struggling ex-boxer. Movie-going audiences at that time apparently identified more strongly with an addict who had a vocation and prospects in life than with marginal individuals who had no prospects. The risk of losing all of his life advantages added dramatic tension to the protagonist's circumstances in the film. Its take-home message about our shared vulnerability was that intelligent, normally industrious people can fall victim to alcoholism and become so impaired that they cannot overcome their addiction without help, a theme that perhaps enhanced the film's impact on its North American audience.

The following year (1947) the movie *Smash Up: The Story of a Woman* starring Susan Hayward was released. Like male drug and alcohol films, it expresses a motif we call "descent into hell," which subsumes other themes under it, including deteriorating lifestyle, abandonment of moral and ethical principles, and obsession with drug procurement. The movie tells the story of a nightclub singer whose career is put on hold as she invests herself in supporting her husband's career (a common enough occurrence during this era). But as his career takes off, hers slides into an addictive relationship with alcohol until she "hits bottom." Four years later, a movie with a similar theme about the threat of alcoholism and its destructive power appeared under the title of *Night into Morning* with Ray Milland. Released about the same time was *Come Fill the Cup*, a movie with an all-star cast (James Cagney, Raymond Massey, Jackie Gleason and Gig Young) that conveyed the message that people with drinking problems must help other people to stay sober themselves. Soon thereafter, came the well-acted and award-winning film *Come Back Little Sheba* starring Burt Lancaster and Shirley Booth. Lancaster plays a man who dropped out of medical school to support a woman he impregnated but did not love. In self-pity, he turns to drinking, which causes him to have bouts of murderous anger. It too reflects the "descent into hell" theme although, in the end, Lancaster's character begins to see the light.

In 1962, the issue of alcoholism received another highly acclaimed treatment in Blake Edwards's *The Days of Wine and Roses*. Like *The Lost Weekend*, *The Days of Wine and Roses* had advantages, including an innovative director, a talented cast, and a great musical score. In fact, its only Academy Award recognized the best original song composed as part of Henry Mancini's score. The film received other nominations, including the co-protagonists played by Jack Lemmon and Lee Remick, art direction, and set design. This version of the alcoholism movie used some structural components of the type we call "young junkies in love" —the more experienced partner introducing the naïve partner to the drug, shared escalation of use, deterioration of life circumstances (job loss, destitution), and abandonment of previously held values. In a departure from other narratives in which both young junkies in love continue their addictive paths to self-destruction, Joe Clay, the male lead in *The Days of Wine and Roses*, withdraws from alcohol addiction, experiences recidivism caused by his unreformed wife, only to withdraw from alcohol again. As the film ends, he comes to the realization that he cannot reconcile with a wife who will not give up alcohol. This ending is not simply a departure from the "young junkies in love" type; it also departs from Hollywood's customary "love conquers all" theme. As with *The Lost Weekend*'s protagonist, Joe Clay is a promising, upper-middle-class professional who begins to lose everything through his constant drinking. Again, this vulnerability of an otherwise bright and capable adult to alcoholic recidivism seemed to resonate with the viewer audiences of 1962. A forceful intervention by his 12-step sponsor (played by Jack Klugman) helped to convince Joe Clay that he could not remain sober if he accepted his wife back in his home, and this action reiterated that alcoholics need help to remain sober, this time in opposition to previously supportive (and enabling) social environments.

In our discussion of high-profile, Oscar-worthy acting performances about addiction, we cannot omit Katharine Hepburn's performance in the movie version of Eugene O'Neill's play, *A Long Day's Journey into Night*. As the morphine-addicted wife of an alcoholic, she took viewers through the biographical cautionary stations of suffering, from the introduction, to addiction, to dysfunction, all in retrospect, as the action involved only a single day. The combination of Hepburn's acting and O'Neill's writing produced what could be called the apogee of films on the human condition of the addict, at least up to 1962. The introduction of Mary Tyrone (Hepburn's character) to morphine involved a different kind of agency. Rather than the often portrayed lover or boyfriend, a physician had introduced Mary to morphine, an example of what is known in the literature as an iatrogenic etiology. Furthermore, Mary's pharmacist and her sons had all worked to enable her continued use, including the concealment of her addiction from her husband. Consequently, she had no experience with the desperate, principle-breaking, morality-bending behavior often portrayed in films that have addiction as a central theme. Nevertheless, O'Neill clearly presented Mary's addiction as an exacerbating factor in dysfunctional household relations. In that sense, *A Long Day's Journey into Night* was consistent with the damage assessments in other addiction movies—addiction makes things worse, much worse. In our own ethnographic research, we have encountered households in which one or more members have been addicts, usually in a poly-drug mode. In all cases, the presence of the addicts was highly disruptive, with impacts on child care, interaction among adults, and even decor (e.g., when the addict sold off articles of furniture to obtain drugs). Research by Linda Bennett and Steven Wolin (1990) has shown that alcoholism in a family member can subsume structure-building family rituals. Their findings (Bennett and Wolin 1990:202) show that "those families whose rituals were most subsumed by the alcoholism ... evidenced a greater incidence of intergenerational continuity of the alcoholism among the grown children ... than those families which kept their family rituals distinct from the alcohol abuse behavior."

Exploitation films have never really died off completely, but most have had production values considerably better than those of *Reefer Madness* or *The Cocaine Fiends*. One film adaptation of a 1966 Jacqueline Suzanne novel clearly belongs in this category—*The Valley of the Dolls* (1967). It was one of the first to dramatize the misuse of prescription medication, focusing primarily on barbiturates. The film's title used a slang term ("dolls") for sedative/hypnotic pills favored by women in show business. Not really focusing on addiction, this movie emphasized the un-glamorous aspects of what appeared to be glamorous lifestyles in which the players were constantly at risk due to their drug use. Suicide was always possible, as the barbiturates on the players' night stands were eminently capable of killing via overdose.[3] Unlike the exploitation films that preceded it, *The Valley of the Dolls* did not moralize over the poor choices made by its principal characters, but rather caused the audience to witness their downfall without comment. At the time of its release, the pills at the center of this film's drug content were about to be supplanted by a new generation of sedative/hypnotics and anxiolytics that were much safer to use than barbiturates.[4] Consequently, the drug content of *Valley of the Dolls* became irrelevant only a year after its release. Its primary source of notoriety was co-star Sharon Tate, who in 1969 fell victim to Charles Manson's gang in a horrific burglary/murder.

Fifteen years after *The Valley of the Dolls,* the next generation of prescription medications received attention in a film entitled *I'm Dancing as Fast as I Can* (1982). Among drug films, this one occupies the space of autobiographical narrative, in which the author, Barbara Gordon, is the protagonist. Most of the other films discussed here are biographical, but not autobiographical, and this may explain the somewhat puzzling portrayal of what would seem to be an exaggeration of the problems associated with Valium. Critical commentary at the time the movie came out expressed confusion about the nature of the protagonist's problems. Literally millions of primary-care physicians at that time were prescribing benzodiazepines (the class of drugs to which Valium belongs) to their patients, often for clearly identified anxiety, but also for a variety of much more vague symptoms. Even when not quite appropriate, most of these prescriptions had little or no aftermath, and certainly did not result in the institutionalization of the recipients. Why, then, was this woman having such severe trouble with Valium? The film never succeeds in explaining the origins of these problems, which include treatment for addiction to Valium and time in a mental hospital. Impairment related to use of Valium is, as the national statistics tell us, a relatively rare occurrence, especially when one considers the immense denominator in that fraction. The Community Epidemiology Work Group reports some emergency department and hotline calls that referred to problems with Valium, but those made up only a small proportion of the benzodiazepine-related problems in reporting cities (CEWG 2011). In 1982, Valium had a larger share of the pool of benzodiazepine misuse than it presently does, because of the emergence of Xanax and Clonipin as favored recreational drugs. Misuse of prescription sedative/hypnotic drugs has otherwise not received much cinematic attention since the release of *I'm Dancing as Fast as I Can.*

Heroin use remained part of the filmmakers' repertoire of topics throughout the 1970s, 1980s, and 1990s, and during that period, the content included two major types, the biographical film and the young junkies in love type. *The Panic in Needle Park* (1971) exemplified the latter type, providing a breathless, unpleasant narrative about young people who become heroin addicts in the big city. The character known as Bobby, played by Al Pacino, and the Helen character, played by Kitty Winn, do not exactly "meet cute," as she is in the process of recuperating from a substandard abortion when he visits her in the hospital after a brief introduction by her former lover (played by Raul Julia). She is the naïve partner who is at first unfamiliar with heroin, but under Bobby's tutelage, she takes it up. The film essentially follows their relationship through the already familiar structure of young junkies in love: plunge into addiction, destitution, prostitution, and loss of previously held values, conflict, betrayal, forgiveness, further betrayal, and expression of desire to escape the sorrowful life they have constructed. Well portrayed are the emotional perils of addiction, including selfishness and self-absorption. This film even has a certain verisimilitude that the other cinematic treatments of addiction that came before it lacked. The absence of a musical score gives the scenes in *The Panic in Needle Park* additional grittiness and harsh tone, especially when Bobby and Helen fight. Other scenes include some of the most explicit images of self-injection ever to appear on screen up to the time of the film's release. Our own observational experience (e.g., Page, Chitwood et al. 1990; Page, Smith and Kane 1990a, 1990b; Simons and Singer 2006) matches the self-injection scenes in *The Panic in Needle Park* somewhat, although use of tourniquet ties was far less frequent in our observations than in the movie, due to our frequent observations of injectors resorting to areas in the body not amenable to tie-off (e.g., neck, behind the knee, between the toes, and some locations on the body trunk).

In 1972, an autobiographical film featured heroin addiction as it occurred in the Great Depression. William Duffy had co-written a memoire with Billie Holiday. Chris Clarke, Suzanne dePasse, and Clarence McCloy adapted this work into a screenplay entitled *Lady Sings the Blues*. The movie starred Diana Ross in the title role, and it had her performing the music of Billie Holiday. Holiday's experience with heroin, according to the screenplay, began as she reacted to the things she saw during a concert tour in the south. She apparently witnessed the aftermath of a lynching, which, besides leading to her choosing and performing a topical song that bemoans lynchings ("Strange Fruit"), made Holiday so depressed that she started using heroin. Because she had a skill and multiple enablers in her immediate social environment, Holiday was able to avoid sinking into criminality or prostitution in order to feed her heroin habit. Nevertheless, she could not avoid arrest for possession of narcotics (Singer and Mirheg 2006). As in the cases of the protagonists in *The Lost Weekend* and *Days of Wine and Roses,* the risk taken by Billie Holiday in using heroin involved an otherwise promising career jeopardized by her addiction, in this instance, to heroin. The film makes the case that Holiday was self-medicating with heroin, as a result of the combined influences of the racist mistreatment received by people of color, strong feelings about what she had seen in the American South, and the presence and availability of heroin among jazz musicians during this era. No doubt, there were also gender discrimination issues that contributed to Holiday's slide into addiction, both in terms of her troubled romantic relationships and in her career.

Although it did not win any Academy Awards, *Lady Sings the Blues* received five nominations. Its box office drawing power was considerably better than any other film that featured principal characters whose heroin use was essential to the plot. It also communicated effectively that black heroin users were especially vulnerable to the enforcement of drug use laws. The heroin withdrawal scenes in *Lady Sings the Blues* recapitulated the vivid sequence of seizures, shakes, and cold sweats shown in other biographical films, further building heroin's reputation for engendering powerful body-wracking withdrawal symptoms. In contrast, *Lenny,* (1974) a film about the life of Lenny Bruce, a white stand-up comic of the 1950s and 1960s, acknowledged his use of illegal drugs, but he became vulnerable to police primarily because of his avant-garde use of profanity on stage. An overdose of morphine killed Bruce in 1966, but the film about his life focused more on his controversial stand-up act than his drug use.

Three years after *Lady Sings the Blues* was released, a sequel to *The French Connection* directed by John Frankenheimer came to North American screens. *The French Connection II* followed the protagonist, Popeye Doyle to Marseilles, and in a truly unusual twist of plot, the drug traffickers kidnapped Doyle and forced repeated injections of heroin on him, making him an addict. After his release by the traffickers, Doyle's character went through a harrowing and histrionic withdrawal experience during which Gene Hackman, the actor portraying Doyle, performed cold sweats, shakes, convulsions, nonsensical gibbering, and general incapacitation in what seemed a compendium of all of the heroin withdrawal scenes that went before *The French Connection II.* Frankenheimer seemed to have set as his objective to portray withdrawal from heroin addiction as the worst experience a human being can have other than death itself, and certainly for people who die peacefully, a much more painful one. The traffickers' purposeful inflicting of addiction on Doyle, leading to his excruciating suffering amplified the film's momentum toward retribution against Alain Charnier, the lead trafficker, and his henchmen. Nevertheless, the viewer wonders whether or not methadone treatment involving gradual downward titration of methadone doses might have eased Doyle's withdrawal experience, as it has done for many thousands of addicts. Frankenheimer and Hackman apparently recognized an opportunity to shoot a dramatic scene that contributed to the film's momentum as it barreled toward Doyle's revenge against his tormentors. Whatever its merit or lack thereof, this film contributed the concept of forced addiction to the cinematic vocabulary of drug use. The concept, in fact, has been operative for years, not in making police detectives miserable, but in the murky world of human trafficking, in which addiction is a tool for enslaving young women who are forced to work as prostitutes as a means of gaining access to drugs.

Three films released in the 1980s recapitulated or presented variants of the "young junkies in love" theme: *Christiane F. —We Children of the Bahnhof Zoo, Sid and Nancy,* and *Drugstore Cowboy. Christiane F.,* released in 1983 with a sound track by David Bowie, who also appears in the movie performing in concert, was a biographical film based on journalist interviews with Vera Christiane Felscherionow. It had the most disturbing premise of the three 1980s young junkies in love films—that children as young as age thirteen could become involved in heroin use and eventually become addicts. The fact that the protagonists were so young, about 13 years old, made *Christiane* especially upsetting for much of its viewing audience. Other than featuring very young addicts, the film followed the "young junkies" trajectory with little divergence: the couple meets in an anarchic club scene; the female partner learns heroin use from the male; they become addicted; they go through harrowing withdrawal symptoms, in this case, together; they become re-addicted; the female resorts to sex work and steals money from her mother to get heroin. In a slight departure from the standard "young junkies" format, the male partner engages in sex work with an older man. Although 13-year-old addicts undoubtedly exist in the midst of large populations of heroin users, most of the data available on injecting drug users indicate that the typical onset of self-injection behavior occurs at about 18 or 19, although non-injection drug use may begin as much as 5 years earlier (McCoy et al. 1979). Therefore, *Christiane F.'s* experience is rather unusual. In fact, it appears that people over 35 are more likely to take up heroin use than people under 17. Nevertheless, this film stimulated much discussion of drug problems in Germany and the rest of Europe. The notion that drugs represent a menace to youth has pervaded much of the cinematic material reviewed here, and this menace seems particularly compelling and frightening if it targets the very young. In the extreme, we have seen the exaggerations of *Reefer Madness* about the vulnerability of tender teens, and the case of Janet Cooke's fabricated newspaper reports describing an eight-year-old addict (McGrath 1981) that garnered considerable public attention thirty years ago. Ms. Cooke's Pulitzer Prize, which she subsequently forfeited, stands as an example of the public's thirst for this kind of story and the superficial credulity of the press when this kind of content appears. *Christiane F.,* in other words, on whose life the film was based, was relatively rare among injecting heroin addicts. As a result of the film's success in Germany, a subculture of teenage girls began to imitate Christine F's clothing style and to hang out at the Bahnhof Zoo station, the central transport facility in Western Berlin during the period when the city was divided. This generated considerable concern among authorities that despite the dreariness of the film *Christiane F.* would become a cult drug-using role model for impressionable youth.

Because so much of it appeared in the press as it was happening, the veracity of *Sid and Nancy* (1986) as a "young junkies in love" story outline was never in doubt. This story of two addicts, Sid Vicious, punk rocker of the Sex Pistols and his girlfriend, Nancy Spungen had all of the major components of "young junkies in love." One taught the other to use heroin (Nancy taught Sid). They fell deeply in love as they became seriously addicted. Sid's relationship with the other members of the Sex Pistols deteriorated until the band broke up. The relationship between Sid and Nancy became increasingly destructive until it culminated in both of their deaths. Key incidents in the romance between Sid and Nancy bracketed the entire arc of the film, which opened in the aftermath of Nancy's fatal stabbing and ended with Sid's fatal overdose, laying out a sequence of retrospective scenes depicting the initiation and development of the pair's troubled love affair. The story of the Sex Pistols' rise and fall as a pioneering punk band hung from the love story's framework. None of the other "young junkies" films has a larger, historical story (the rise of the Sex Pistols) that depended for its exposition on the central love story. *Sid and Nancy* rivaled any of the others in the intense unpleasantness of scenes in which the addicted couples are alone together.

Drugstore Cowboy (1989) was much more picaresque in tone than any of the films about addiction that preceded it. The protagonist and his girlfriend recapitulated the principal features of "young junkies in love," but as irresponsible white young people whose primary motivation was to get high and stay high at the expense of pharmacies, they gave the whole homologous arc of their story a sardonic edge that seemed new and different. Based on an autobiographical book by James Fogle, the film followed the protagonist, played by Matt Dillon, as he assembled a crew that set off to burglarize as many pharmacies as necessary to satisfy their need to get high. Set in the Pacific Northwest, the film had the band of drug thieves involved in misadventures that seemed comical and cautionary at the same time. When one of the band died, the tone changed drastically, not just because of the horror of death, but because the group began to understand the seriousness of their activities. Bob Hughes, the protagonist, decided to abandon the group's drug-driven lifestyle at that point in the movie, inevitably encountering further difficulties and eventual incarceration.

Toward the end of the film, author and noted lifelong drug user William S. Burroughs, as Tom, a wizened longtime junkie, held forth on the injustice of government policies against drug use and expressed his own defiant advocacy for getting high however he chooses. The entire film communicated a kind of ambivalent attitude about drug use, North American drug laws, and the consequences of a drug-oriented lifestyle. The filmmakers obviously recognize that there are consequences for illegal drug use, but they appear to question whether or not these consequences primarily are constructed by the legal context in which drug use occurs. Tom's/Burroughs's soliloquy would argue for the latter conclusion, but other parts of the movie appear to caution the viewer that death may be an outcome for this kind of behavior. Our experience as anthropological researchers has involved, among other activities, many long conversations with drug users, both individually and in focus groups (e.g., Singer et al. 2001; Singer 2006). Those conversations, in which drug users and addicts discussed in depth their long-term relationship with drugs, affirm the duality of addiction as expressed in *Drugstore Cowboy,* that use of drugs can hold great wonders for some, but its risks can at any time overtake the user. In the end, most street drug users we have interviewed come to despise themselves for the damaging choices they have made and hold, at best, ambivalent attitudes about drugs. There are parallels between how some drug users talk about their addiction and the agonizing narratives of tenacious but unrequited lovers.

Besides introducing the international movie-going public to Ewan Mc-Gregor, *Trainspotting* (1996) jarred film audiences with its unique combination of humor, horror, arresting images, and almost prankish turns of plot. In terms of structure, it did not bother with most of the conventions of how film had portrayed addiction and its process. In the film's first few minutes, the protagonist (Renton, played by McGregor) is an already-established heroin addict, willing to plunge into the world's most squalid toilet to retrieve opioid suppositories bought as a final dose before withdrawing from heroin. Rather than showing the audience how Renton acquired his addiction, *Trainspotting* practically began its narrative by showing how he went about preparing to withdraw from heroin. Renton's preparations for the withdrawal experience included the collection of an array of paraphernalia, including food, buckets for waste, Valium, television, print pornography, and music (Boyd 2008:94) and nailing the door of his cheap hotel room shut with him inside. Tommy, a minor character, took up heroin use in the course of the film, eventually contracting AIDS and dying. Allison, another minor character with already-established addiction and a baby to care for, allowed the baby to die of neglect, one of the most upsetting and drug-user-damning sequences in the film. Renton went through withdrawal twice during the course of the film, the first time in a light-hearted mood. The second withdrawal included the physical paroxysms often shown in other films, with the addition of some truly bizarre hallucinations depicting Allison's deceased baby crawling across the ceiling.

Trainspotting presented the most wildly varied view of addiction ever on film, up to the date of its release. When Renton explains the attraction of heroin, he offers the following description of the heroin "rush": "Take the best orgasm you've ever had, multiply it by a thousand, and you're still nowhere near it" (Boyd 2008:96). On the other hand, the same character described in detail the suffering he and others in this life endured as consequences of either personal or parental addiction. Tommy died of AIDS, Spud spent time in prison, and most horrifyingly, Baby Dawn died of neglect as the adults around her binged on drugs. Some controversy emerged when *Trainspotting* was released because it seemed to have too sympathetic a view of heroin use and addiction. In contrast, Boyd (2008:98) points out that no heroin user appeared in the film who was not either addicted or formerly addicted. Boyd also recognizes that *Trainspotting* presented addiction to heroin as a temporary condition that the main characters took on or shed according to their psychological states. This quality of temporariness seems at odds with Tom's assessment of addiction in *Drugstore Cowboy* during which he repeats the common phase about drug users, "once a junkie, always a junkie." Our own research over years of observing, hanging out with, and interviewing heroin and other injecting-drug users testifies to the intense duality of addiction, which can be temporary, and in the strictest sense, under control of the users, but also tends to frequent recidivism (cf. McCoy et al 1979; Page 1997; Page and Salazar 1997; Singer 1994; 2006). In truth, addicts can withdraw from heroin when they please, with or without assistance, and usually the withdrawal is perceived as worth it because going through the treatment process places the habit under better control, making it less demanding on the users. Furthermore, for a time after withdrawal, returning users get more pleasure from the drug than they did before withdrawal, when their tolerance for their drug of choice was high.

Another film that used humor to depict the plight of the addict who wants to quit, *Gridlock'd* (1997), played to a limited audience, but made key points about the barriers to access faced by addicts, even when they overdose. The central characters, Spoon (played by Tupac Shakur in one of his few film appearances), Stretch (Tim Roth), and Cookie (Thandie Newton), shared with biographical film protagonists, as in *Lady Sings the Blues* and *Ray,* the characteristic that they had talent, and, like Mark Renton in *Trainspotting,* they had the good sense to decide to kick heroin when faced with potential severe consequences. The comedy in *Gridlock'd* emerged from their attempts, first to deal with an acute situation, in which Cookie overdosed and

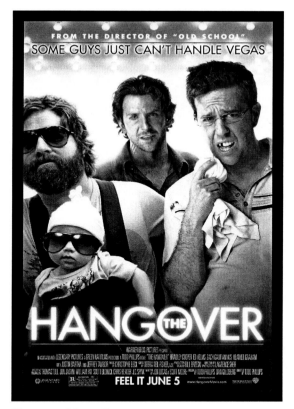

Hangover Movie Poster

Stretch and Spoon tried to get an ambulance to come pick her up, and second when they tried to gain acceptance into a drug-treatment program. In the first situation, after being brushed aside by the 911 operator, they called in again and told 911 that they were under attack and that a white woman had been shot. Although they thought this story would get immediate results, with extra police cars, the ambulance did not come, and the pair was forced to take their friend to the hospital themselves. Again, after failed attempts to gain admission to drug treatment, Spoon and Stretch devised a plan in which one (Stretch, who was already shot) stabbed the other in order to gain admission to a hospital for both of them. This last-ditch strategy apparently succeeded. *Gridlock'd* avoided showing any of the rigors of withdrawal, and ended by suggesting that all three of the central characters, Cookie, Spoon, and Stretch had apparently withdrawn successfully from heroin and were playing happily in their band.

The odyssey of these two "buddies" took the audience through the often baffling and always frustrating process of confronting bureaucracies as experienced by addicts. In our own experience as street-drug researchers, we have come to realize that treatment centers often establish policies aimed at only admitting those addicts who have good presumption of success. In one of the most blatant examples of this kind of policy, a cocaine injector who was interested in receiving treatment laboriously (due to his hip injuries) walked several blocks from his home to the center that urged him to come in for treatment. Upon arrival, the screeners told him to come back in a week to "make sure he was serious about treatment." Of course, they never saw him again. Repeatedly, our study participants have expressed the impression that treatment centers do not really want them to come in for treatment. One of the ways this is sometimes manifest is in having policies that work well for institutions but poorly for their drug-involved patients, such as refusal to recognize that drug users can have romantic relationships (like other people) or that having children is a primary reason some drug users do not enter or, if they enter, stay in treatment (because they are concerned about what is happening to their children). *Gridlock'd* demurred at the prospect of portraying withdrawal pangs one more time, perhaps because the filmmaker did not believe the previously depicted hyperboles of *The Man with the Golden Arm* or *Lady Sings the Blues*. Its unique success lay in its sardonic, but generally accurate assertions about the deep flaws of the health-care system in the United States, especially in the system's interactions with poor and working class clientele, and that clientele's dependence on emergency care (Singer 1994). Moreover, the film affirms an important aspect of our current treatment apparatus—that it participates in the construction of the drug-using Other and acts accordingly.

Requiem for a Dream (2000) used multiple story lines to focus on both the nature of addiction in its various forms and the dysfunctionality of a society that produces so many ways of being dependent on drugs. Its story lines include a "junky buddies" pair whose addiction, in the tradition of biographical cautionary tales, led to nightmarish outcomes, including amputation and prison-based abuse. In a tangential "young junkies in love" plot line, Marion, the girlfriend of one of the buddies, was cajoled and eventually forced into the sex trade in order to obtain drugs for the couple. Sarah, the mother of one of the buddies had a quiz-show addiction that led to a diet-pill addiction as she prepared to appear on a quiz show for which she qualified. Critical commentary on *Requiem for a Dream* expressed some skepticism about the terrible ends to which the main characters plummeted, noting that the director seemed to take pleasure in devastating people whom he set up initially as decent, sympathetic folks (Boyd 2008:99). This approach to cinematic treatment of addiction is especially reminiscent of the "disposable" characters in *Cocaine Fiends* and *Reefer Madness*, as *Requiem for a Dream* left its characters irredeemably crushed. Our own experience leads us to comment that, in long-term interaction with street-based addicts and non-addicted drug users, we seldom encountered people who lacked resilience, even if that resilience only led to recidivistic addiction. Whatever the addiction, even in the face of consequential disease, such as hepatitis C and AIDS, participants in our studies usually have been capable of recuperation, humor, and to varying degrees, redemption. No small number of them, however, die as a direct or indirect result of their involvement with drugs (Singer et al. 2000). Death of drug users comes in many forms, including disease, overdose, violence, exposure, automobile accidents, and fires.

The year 2000 also saw the release of a film that had a large budget, a heavyweight cast, with a sweeping point of view about drug use in the United States and its logistic partner Mexico. The movie, *Traffic*, featured Michael Douglas, Benicio del Toro, Don Cheadle, Catherine Zeta-Jones, Topher Grace, James Brolin, Erika Christensen, and Amy Irving, among others, and was directed by Steven Soderbergh. Its arenas of action included parts of Mexico (Tijuana, Sonora) and the borderland areas of the United States Southwest; Cincinnati, Ohio; Washington, DC; and San Diego and Los Angeles, California. Because he changed venues in the final cut of the film so often, Soderbergh gave each place a tint of its own (e.g., sepia for Mexico, bluish gray for Cincinnati). The parts of this film that focused on addiction to heroin involved a well-to-do young girl and her friends, a feature that is actually rare, but fit well into the overall story line. Caroline Wakefield's pathway into addiction began in the company of bored, cynical young people looking for exciting things to do in Cincinnati and deciding that smoking heroin was the ticket to adventure. As we have said elsewhere, high-school age youth seldom resort to heroin injection,[5] but rather graduate to it. In this case, because Caroline Wakefield's father Robert (played by Michael Douglas) is the newly designated director of the Office of National Drug Control Policy (ONDCP), her acquisition of an addiction to heroin is absolutely essential to the story of that office. Robert Wakefield's journey into the role of parent of an addict ultimately led him to question the US policy on the War on Drugs. After he had the experience of discovering Caroline's addiction, finding her in desperate straits, and enrolling her in treatment, he addressed a gathering in Washington in his capacity as director of the ONDCP by asking the question, "How can we declare war on ourselves?" His realization that the "War on Drugs" sets drug users against non-users as adversaries within our "United States" brings into focus the futility of engaging in such a "war." The movie, however, had little impact on the prosecution of that multibillion dollar war, which continues even though it still fails to achieve its ostensible goals. In part, this is so because advocates of this war continue (somehow) to convince a distressed public that it is not, in fact, a war on ourselves, but rather on a group of nefarious others.

Boyd (2008:137–138), vehemently criticizes *Traffic* on grounds of racism, for depicting the venal and corrupt drug traffickers as Mexican. According to Boyd, the scenes in which Robert Wakefield tracks Caroline down to a black drug dealer's apartment also reflects the filmmaker's racism. This criticism is at odds with nearly all of the critical commentary on the film, which eventually won Golden Globes and Academy Awards, and various film-critic awards, notably including Soderbergh for best director and Del Toro for best supporting actor. We point out, first of all, that the most sympathetic character in the entire film is Javier, Del Toro's character, who is portrayed as Mexican. We also note that none of the actions of the Mexican cartel leaders and henchmen are exaggerated in the least, based on what is known about drug traffic across the US border with Mexico. Furthermore, we have seen repeatedly in our own work that when a white drug user of either sex is seeking safe haven from parents and/or police, the predominantly black neighborhood is where they go to find safe houses, people willing to take them in, availability of drugs, and a generally nonjudgmental attitude about their drug use. This does not mean that black neighborhoods are dominated by drug dealers and users—far from it. The majority of these neighborhoods' inhabitants avoid drug use or traffic, but those houses where drug use occurs tend to avoid revealing their activities to neighbors (cf. Page and Llanusa-Cestero 2006). In that low-profile setting, a white person can hide out and count on the discretion of the hosts. Caroline's predicament in the Cincinnati ghetto is a reflection of the realities of drug use in many parts of the United States, not a function of racism on the part of the filmmaker. More importantly, it is a reflection of where society tolerates drug sales and use, the role minority neighborhoods play in servicing of the vices of suburban whites, and the utility of drug scenes in minority neighborhoods in anchoring stereotypes about drug users in society.

Boyd (2008) may have been disturbed by the large-scale processes that produce drug traffic, addiction, and drug enforcement. Those processes are incontestably racist, and have much to do with how addiction is described and perceived in public discourse. The gratuitously manipulative and quasi-racist parts of the Weatherly segments in *Traffic* involve the sex trade that Caroline uses to obtain drugs. In the film, Soderbergh made it look as though the black drug dealer had simply taken advantage of a white girl in trouble, but in fact, white women in a predominantly black environment may use their sexual allure to obtain the drugs they want and need. He may have been guilty of presenting exploitation in only one direction. We find it difficult to envision a presentation of Soderbergh's material through re-alignment of ethnicities and racial categories. Drug traffic through Canada, although present, is far less of an issue than traffic through Mexico. With regard to the presence of inner-city ghettoes and their identification with drug use and drug traffic, very few cities in North America do not have that dynamic in place, even though people of color in the United States use drugs less than the white non-Hispanic population (Wallace and Murdoff 2002, Substance Abuse and Mental Health Services Administration 2008). The image of ghetto as haven for drug traffic and use, we contend, is a function of its exploitable position as economically disadvantaged. Bourgois made this point (1997, 1998) in explaining the adaptive choices present in ghetto settings. To illustrate the exploitative nature of the ghetto environment, Topher Grace's character explains to Judge Weatherly that drug markets exist in black neighborhoods for the convenience of white drug users. Moreover, left out of most depictions like this are sectors that ultimately are part of the global drug trade, such as the role of "respectable" banks in the laundering of drug money. In his song "Jokerman," Bob Dylan proclaims "Steal a little, they throw you in jail; steal a lot and they make you a king." The truth of this assertion is seen in a *Guardian* newspaper commentary that accurately observes "global banks are the financial services wing of drug cartels" (Vulliamy 2008). Notably, for example, Britain's largest bank, HSBC was fined $1.9 billion dollars for its role in money laundering for Mexican drug groups like the Sinaoloa illicit drug-smuggling company. While the bank admitted to violating the Banking Secrecy Act and The Trading with the Enemy Act, despite these serious violations, no corporate leaders from HSBC were sent to prison, a punishment routinely administered to individuals charged with the possession of small amounts of marihuana. The HSBC incident is not an isolated case. Two years earlier, Wachovia was fined $50 million and made to turn over $11 million in drug money. In the Wachovia case, a whistle blower working for the bank who exposed its illegal activities was fired for attempting to alert his supervisors about the bank's money laundering (although he did win a law suit for unfair dismissal). As with HSBC, no one from Wachovia went to jail. In contrasting the treatment of often poor minority drug users with that of generally wealthy white money launderers we see the real face of racism in the world of illicit drugs.

Perhaps the most searing and difficult-to-watch piece of filmmaking about drug addiction so far in the 21st century is *Dope Sick Love,* a documentary shown by Home Box Office in 2005. The camera follows two opioid-addicted couples through their cyclical efforts to avoid the symptoms of withdrawal from drugs and derive whatever pleasure they can from the effects of the drugs they buy. The couples' repertoires for what drug researcher Michael Agar would call "copping" (procuring drugs) include appeals to parents to wire cash, petty thievery, and even robbery. Their round of activities is frenetic, as every four hours or so, the symptoms of withdrawal are bound to return. Activities have a frantic pace, especially as each cycle closes in, making the couples impatient, irascible, and increasingly desperate. When they have secured the needed "dope," the couples' movements are swift and practiced, and their self-injection routines are very efficient. Throughout the film, the camera operator's eye for detail gives viewers access to the minutiae of drug-taking behavior, including use of public toilets as a source of water, exclusive use of plastic diabetic syringes, use of mouth and teeth for handling syringes, and lighting and handling of crack pipes among many other details. These activities all strongly resemble the behaviors we have witnessed in natural settings as part of our research, with one notable exception: the ease with which these injectors locate and "hit" (i.e., inject into) veins. In our experience, this process can be laborious, time consuming, and painful, primarily because among long-term experienced self-injectors, many of their "best" peripheral veins are no longer accessible, due to collapse caused by over-use (Page, Smith and Kane 1990b). The almost-balletic efficiency of the dope sick lovers does not ring true in that sense, perhaps because the process of finding veins has the advantage of film editing. A recent dissertation completed by Jennifer Syvertsen (2012) presents a very different view of lovers injecting each other. Based on hours of observation and open-ended interviews with couples who inject together, the combination of mutual concern, love, sexual desire, addiction, and pain receives excruciating attention in this work's narratives.

To dismiss *Candy* (2006) as a re-hash of the *Days of Wine and Roses* would give short shrift to fine acting by Heath Ledger, Geoffrey Rush, and Abbie Cornish, who have major roles in this creatively conceived Australian film. Although it followed the "young junkies in love" trajectory closely, *Candy* placed a framework around the standard processes of meeting, charming each

other, teaching how to shoot heroin, compromising personal values, prostitution, thievery, withdrawal, recidivism, betrayal, and ultimately, separation.
The first phase, during which the partners plunged into love and addiction
simultaneously, was titled, taking a hint from Dante Allighieri, "Heaven." The
second phase, in which the lovers moved into a period of having to maintain
each other's habits, was called "Earth." The film maker, Neil Armfield, chose
to call the final phase of the junkie lovers' lives "Hell," as they attempted to
live together, first using methadone, and finally detoxified. They eventually
discovered that heroin was what had tied their lives together in the first place,
and that realization led to their permanent separation.

We included this film in our review primarily because it was the only
Australian film that focused on addiction. In addition, however, in terms of
production values and overall quality, the film certainly meets the standards
of the Australian film-making tradition, which has shown vitality and creativity, and this level of quality places *Candy* on a par with North American
and British films focused on addiction, such as *The Panic in Needle Park* and
Trainspotting. It also covers a variety of addict that has received attention in
movies in terms of alcohol, rather than illegal street drugs—the middle class
addict. The two lovers began their descent by cadging "loans" from friends
and family, and eventually resorting to crime in order to feed their habits,
but their lifestyles had none of the gritty character that dominated *The Panic
in Needle Park* or *The Man with the Golden Arm*. Furthermore, the hell that
eventually emerged from the couple's addiction was not the obvious abyss
of slavery to a drug, but the hell of realizing that what they thought to be
durable love had been held together by addiction, and without addiction, it
lacked a foundation. The lovers in *Days of Wine and Roses* came to a similar
conclusion when the Joe Clay character rejected his wife's overture to get back
together, realizing that she had no intention of quitting drinking. This kind
of ending reinforces the middle class value that sobriety must supersede all
other priorities, including love between man and woman, which otherwise
is celebrated in film as one of the core values of society. This review hardly
addressed all of the films that have been produced with drug use as a core
theme. New movies, from big productions like *Flight* (2012), in which Den-
zel Washington portrays a hard-drinking, heavy drug using and reckless
airplane pilot, to lower budget, less-well-known films like *Lost in the Crack*
(2012) (titled *Purgatory* during production), staring Rob Lutz, about the life
of a drug addict and other characters caught in what film advertisements
described as "a perfect storm of tragedy," of course, continue to be made.
This is to be expected because drug use remains an unresolved and thorny

issue in society, and drug users stand as outsiders to the mainstream, objects of curiosity and dread.

TELEVISION SERIES

The television series has some advantages over the feature film in terms of the temporal space it can occupy. Because it consists of one-hour segments that span as many as 25 hours in the course of a season, the television drama can present characters in all of their complexity, ambiguousness, and frailty. The series can also spend time defining the cultural context in which the action occurs. On the topic of addiction, two television series have distinguished themselves in the delineation of their characters and their portrayal of addiction's fraught cultural context: *The Wire* and *Breaking Bad*. In neither case were the protagonists addicts, but in both cases screenplays with well-drawn lesser characters gave the shows' writers ample opportunity to make statements about addiction and its consequences. In *The Wire,* that character was Reginald "Bubbles" Cousins, played by Andre Royo. The Jesse character played by Aaron Paul in *Breaking Bad,* almost a co-protagonist, is a person at the edge of addiction, and his social activities give the audience an up-close

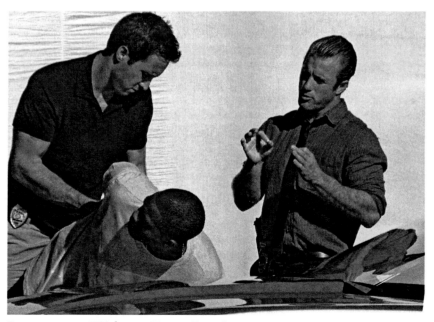

Drug arrest on T.V drama Hawaii Five-O

view of addicts and drug producers nested within the cultural contexts in which they live.

The Wire had admirable structure in its portrayal of an entire system of managing drugs from various points of view, including the street drug user, street drug dealers, higher level drug suppliers, street police, police administrators, federal law enforcement officials, the mayor's office, and the governor's office. Bubbles interacted with parts of this structure as customer to the street-level dealers, informant to the police, and constituent to the mayor. His daily efforts to keep himself supplied with drugs and stay away from the police gave viewers a sense of how the drug system of Baltimore redistributed wealth in favor of the drug dealers and continued to operate despite attempts by street-level police to enforce laws against drugs. Because our own ethnographic experience has tended to focus on people like Bubbles, we found that The Wire's treatment of his character achieved an accurate and humane perspective on the life of an addict. Because we do this kind of work with an eye toward the structural implications of what happens to people like Bubbles, the social panoramic view provided by The Wire had for us an analytic weight seldom seen in television dramas.

Breaking Bad had a different, less structural approach to placing the addict into social context, but it succeeded in establishing an atmosphere of disorganization and deterioration that characterizes many venues where we have seen drugs consumed. Jesse's house, during a period of meth-smoking abandon, became populated with people who were present only for the drugs to be had, and in a matter of days, they converted an orderly house into a squalid mess. We have spent time as drug ethnographers in places like Jesse's living room, and those scenes impressed us as highly authentic. The only things missing from this scene were the offensive smells of stale tobacco, dried urine, and unchecked body odor, which would have made it completely life like. Even more so were some of the places inhabited by minor characters, such as a meth-addicted couple who had stolen an ATM and a character who had received stolen methamphetamine. The interiors of these settings spoke of the director's attention to detail, with their piles of unwashed clothes, scattered defunct appliances, and gaunt, spent inhabitants. The presence of a severely neglected child in the house of the ATM thieves added poignancy to a disturbing view of the human condition in the thrall of addiction to methamphetamine.

Breaking Bad also took a turn at "young junkies in love" as a sub-plot. In season two, Jesse moved into a duplex in which his neighbor (and putative landlady) Jane Margolis (played by Krysten Ritter) was a recovering heroin addict. In this case, both young lovers had prior experience with addiction, and their relationship resulted in relapse for both. Because they were both young, white, from middle-class backgrounds, and very attractive, the characters in this subplot presented a different view of addicts' lifestyles than those presented elsewhere in *Breaking Bad* (e.g., the ATM thieves, the guardian of the stash, or the members of Jesse's crew). Rather than getting into trouble because they did not have enough money, they got into trouble because they had too much money and therefore, too much access to heroin. This condition also contrasted sharply with the lives of addict couples portrayed in *The Panic in Needle* Park and *Christiane F.* Rather than turning tricks at the local strolls to obtain heroin, Jesse and Jane went to art museums. Nevertheless, despite their advantages, the lovers' romance was equally doomed.

Jane's father Donald Margolis (played by John DeLancey) became a tragic figure in *Breaking Bad*'s second season as he imposed rules of conduct and attempted monitoring his daughter's behavior. None of his efforts had any influence on the events, yet he struggled to the end to help his daughter overcome her addiction. His role was akin to that of the classic Greek protagonists, struggling against forces beyond his power to control. The entire viewing audience knew that despite his best efforts, things would "break bad," especially because they had seen Jane conspire to obtain a seemingly endless supply of heroin, claiming that she and Jesse would have one final night with the drug before fleeing to a different life elsewhere. This particular representation of addiction and its consequences is perhaps more relevant to the national structure of the drug market than whatever happens in ghettos and barrios, because the young, white addicts, often from privileged backgrounds, are the ones who drive the market into its multibillion dollar order of magnitude (cf. Chapter 1).

CONCLUSIONS

Interactions between pictorial media and the public can reasonably be expected to have outcomes. On the theme of addiction, the content and tone of pictorial representations have tended toward cautionary tales, intended on some level to warn the public against the lurking dangers of becoming addicted to drugs. Nevertheless, consumption of drugs continues. In the United States, for example, estimates of the total illegal drug traffic exceed $100 billion. The two most lethal (and yet legal) addictive drugs, alcohol and tobacco, account for more billions of dollars in legal production, traffic, and sales. Surveys on how films and television shows have influenced the consumption of mind-altering drugs have yet to be implemented, but clearly, the cautionary messages in films and television have gone largely unheeded by a substantial segment of the US population. If anything, for some, especially youth, the role of drugs in films has served to arouse interest, a pattern found among youth from both developed and underdeveloped countries.

On the other hand, how these media represent addicts and addiction may have exerted sufficient influence on political behavior to have helped to shape laws prohibiting the production, trafficking, and consumption of illegal drugs. *Reefer Madness,* with all of its fabrication, exaggeration, and disinformation, had a lasting impact on the attitudes and perceptions of millions of North Americans with regard to marihuana. Repeated depictions of the throes of withdrawal and the loss of moral compass experienced by people who become addicted to heroin or cocaine made these drugs especially frightening to the viewing public. These pictorial representations emphasized the Otherness of drug users, especially the addicts, and they made addiction seem an inevitable consequence of ever trying heroin or cocaine. The worst of the representations, such as *Reefer Madness* or *The Speed That Kills* treated their main characters as lost souls whose encounters with drugs led to their inescapable destruction. Even films of much higher quality, however, (e.g., *The Panic in Needle Park, The Man with the Golden Arm,* or *Christiane F.*) contributed to the image of addicts as somehow alien, with incomprehensible impulses, and an absence of loyalty to other human beings when they are in the grip of addiction. Stigma naturally follows this kind of demonic characterization, as people internalize the features of drug addicts that make them objects of both fear and fascination. To the viewer, addicts have completely dedicated their lives to one pursuit only—the next dose. The kind of life perceived by the viewers has dual valences. On one hand, it is a form of slavery to one single thing, mind-altering drugs; on the other hand, it liberates the individual (in their own mind at least) from all other social obligations and responsibilities. The latter component, release from everyday social accountability, has a kind of panache for some viewers, while others dismiss voluntary servitude and abdication of all interpersonal obligations in favor of the selfish and self-indulgent pursuit of drugs as something not quite conscionable, indeed, not quite human.

This review and exploration of pictorial representations of addiction attempts to make sense of a series of phenomena that in fact have had ambiguous effects on the viewing publics exposed to them. The diversity of a mass audience, such as that attracted by films and television, assures that the interpretations of presented material will be varied. Unfortunately, the impact of *Reefer Madness* and its disinformation is still palpable in the laws against marihuana use, possession, production, and sale. On the whole, the films discussed above tend to reinforce in a highly visual way the ultimate uselessness of drug users in society. Fortunately, the finely textured and nuanced representations in films and TV series like *The Lost Weekend, Candy,* and *The Wire,* among others, have a chance of contributing to counteracting reductionist and stigmatizing representations of addicts and addictions in the days to come.

NOTES

1 During the last 40 years, Page has spent hundreds of hours in the company of long-term marihuana users, and he has found none of them to be zombie-like in appearance or behavior (cf. Page and Carter 1980; Page 1983; Page, Fletcher, and True 1988).

2 Between 1930 and 1968, the MPAA assigned to all motion pictures a code that certified them under its guidelines for acceptable content.

3 The effective dose to lethal dose ratios for most barbiturates (sodium pentathol, phenobarbital, Seconal, secobarbital, Tuinal) is less than 1:20, making them highly likely to be used for suicide attempts.

4 Non-barbiturate sedatives such as methaqualone were about to be introduced in 1968, and some benzodiazepines (e.g. Librium, Valium, Tranxene, Dalmane, and Xanax) were on the verge of FDA approval. All of these had much higher effective dose to lethal dose ratios than the barbiturates.

5 Some injecting drug use may have been on the rise among adolescents, as indicated in the review by Hopfer et al. (2002) and studies by Fuller et al. (2002) and Miller et al. (2006). Nevertheless, because injecting drug use itself is not widespread, that practice among adolescents, particularly young adolescents, is likely to be relatively rare.

CHAPTER SIX

The Legal Construction of Drug Users

Policy, the Courts, Incarcerating Institutions,
Police Practice, and the War on Drugs

T he United States has possibly the most convoluted, racially biased, and historically fragile policies regarding drug use and drug users of any national polity that assumes the rule of law. This chapter examines this policy structure and its implementation with concerns about the role racial prejudice, the ignoring of the best available science, the impact of how incarceration is applied, its expression in the War on Drugs in practice versus the War on Drugs as ideology, and the use of stereotypes about drug users to perpetuate policies laden with errors in judgment (Windsor and Dunlap 2010). Ultimately, policies and their application comprise the compelling forces that render drug users enemies of society and treat them accordingly. Moreover, the law functions to make drug users available and useful for an array of social purposes. Our fundamental approach to drug laws and associated policy decisions is to interpret them, in part, as exercises in xenophobia, and we use this approach to delineate the relationship between the legislators' perceptions of drug users and the nature and severity of the actual control efforts and punishments that they impose on drug users. At the same time, we are concerned with the ways laws and policies create social and economic uses for those deemed useless.

HISTORY OF POLICY—PROHIBITION: THE MOVEMENT AND THE REALITY.

The 19th century in the United States saw the beginnings of a massive social experiment in prohibiting the consumption of one drug—alcohol. Given the daunting task of achieving ratification in two-thirds of the states, it is astonishing that such a measure could become an amendment to the Constitution. Nevertheless, prohibitionists mustered sufficient public animus and political clout to achieve this action by the federal government.

The Social Value of Drug Addicts: The Uses of the Useless, by Merrill Singer and J. Bryan Page, 153–180.

Historical research suggests that state interest in alcohol consumption has undergone at least three identifiable phases. Preindustrial attention was primarily fueled by a fiscal motivation, alcohol being viewed as taxable commodity. With industrialization and the emergence of laborers as a distinct social class, this attitude was joined and eventually superseded by a concern with temperance. Originally, temperance ideology was a feature of self-discipline in the upper class, but at the turn of the 20th century there emerged a growing alarm about the negative impact of drinking on industrial efficiency and employer control of the working class. Not surprisingly, the main target of the prohibition movement was the drinking practices of working people. Johnson's account of the temperance movement in Rochester, New York, during the 1820s reveals that an intense class struggle ensued around the issue of alcohol consumption.

> Temperance propaganda promised masters social peace, a disciplined and docile labor force and an opportunity to assert moral authority over their men. The movement enjoyed widespread success among the merchants and masters who considered themselves respectable.... Temperance men talked loudest in 1828 and 1829, years in which the autonomy of working-class neighborhoods grew at a dizzying rate.... Wage earners ... now ... drank only in their own neighborhoods and only with each other, and in direct defiance of their employers (Johnson 1978:81–82).

Following the Second World War, the state position toward alcohol consumption again shifted, allowing and supporting the emergence of a highly concentrated alcohol industry with the political muscle to have significant influence on government policy. The current state approach to alcohol consumption has been summarized by Makela and co-workers, based on a review of the alcohol-control policies of eight industrialized nations:

> In general, the State continues to pursue restrictive policies in the non-commercial sector of both manufacture and distribution of alcoholic beverages, whereas the approach toward the commercial segment of the market has become less restrictive and more supportive. In alcohol control, this has taken the form of the opening up of alcohol retail to market pressures and the suppression of non-commercial production (Makela et al. 1981:84).

The character of the pro-industry state bias has been described in an investigation of the political economy of the California wine industry. The state was found to have played a substantial role in the development of monopoly marketing procedures and monopoly-dominated trade associations. By helping to secure the interests of the largest grape growers, state intervention contributed to driving smaller farms out of production: "This new hybrid of private and state power was called agribusiness" (Bunce 1979:49).

Another glimpse at the role of the state in this arena can be seen by examining the activities of the International Center for Alcohol Policies (ICAP). According to its mission statement, the purpose of the ICAP is twofold: (1) to help reduce the abuse of alcohol worldwide and promote understanding of the role of alcohol in society, and (2) to encourage dialogue and pursue partnerships involving the beverage-alcohol industry, the public-health community, and others interested in alcohol policy. At first glance, the ICAP would seem to be a nonprofit scholarly association concerned about the problems of alcohol abuse. In fact, it was established and given its initial $2 million a year operating budget by 11 titans of the global alcohol industry at the time of its founding, including Allied Domecq, Bacardi-Martini, Brown-Forman Beverages, Coors Brewing Company, Foster's Brewing Group Ltd., Guinness, Heineken, IDV, Miller Brewing Co., Joseph E. Seagram & Sons, South African Breweries, and Worldwide. While a pattern of mergers and buyouts has occurred in subsequent years (leading to a steady parade of name changes), these companies came to be well known to public-health advocates as pioneers in the targeted marketing of alcohol to the poor, young, and addicted in the developing world and as opponents of public-health prevention initiatives. Typical of the work of the ICAP (2012) is the production of the study entitled "Producers, Sellers, and Drinkers: Studies of Noncommercial Alcohol in Nine Countries." While ostensibly an investigation of the informal sector of alcohol production and consumption, the underlying messages of the study are revealed in the opening sentences:

> A significant proportion of all alcohol consumed globally is not reflected in official statistics, such as production, trade, and sales figures. These beverages fall into the general category referred to here as "noncommercial" alcohol. The term was chosen in order to differentiate these beverages from alcohol drinks that are produced legally according to set standards, are regulated, and are sold commercially and legally (ICAP 2012:3).

As the choice of words, especially in the last sentence suggests, affirming the legality, high standards, and government-regulated status (in the interest of the public good) of commercial (i.e., the corporate-controlled arena of alcoholic commodities) is certainly an important subtext of this study. This reading is supported by descriptions of the harmful effects, proposal for eradication, role of corruption in the existence of the noncommercial sector and similar linkages of "noncommercial" (which, given the fact that it is often produced to be sold, is a misnomer) with criminality and threats to health.

The parent company of IDV (now UDV), Grand Metropolitan (now Diageo, which owns Burger King and Pillsbury), for example, aggressively promoted José Cuervo in the Islamic country of Malaysia using its "Lick, shoot, suck" promotion in which male drinkers were encouraged to lick salt from a woman's breasts, take a shot of the tequila, then suck from the lime she holds in her mouth. Bacardi-Martini touted its Benedictine D.O.M. (which is almost 40% alcohol) in Malaysia claiming it had "health-enhancing" powers for new mothers.

In Great Britain, Allied Domecq, Bacardi-Martini, and Diageo are all members of The Portman Group, which, although claiming to be concerned solely with the social responsibility issues surrounding alcohol in order to inform public opinion and policy, actively opposed a British attempt to prevent drunk driving by lowering the legal blood-alcohol level for drivers. The Portman Group was found to be offering money to academics to write anonymous critical reviews of the volume *Alcohol Policy and the Public Good*, a book that was written by an international panel of alcohol researchers to provide the scientific foundation for the World Health Organization European Alcohol Action Plan. In Europe, Seagram, Allied Lyons, and Heineken belong to The Amsterdam Group, which sought to take court action against France's policies banning the televising of sports events featuring alcohol advertising. Notably, in 1998, ICAP was able to recruit the US Center for Substance Abuse Prevention (CSAP) to co-issue a report that questions everything from the damaging effects of binge drinking to the causal relationship between alcohol and crime. Noted in the report is recognition that "linking anything with drugs is a way of demonizing it." Thus, expressing an alcohol-industry perspective, the jointly issued report states:

> Perhaps the only simple answer to the question whether alcohol is a drug, is an incomplete one: "Yes, but...." Much more to the point is the subsidiary "Why does it matter?"

In this paper, we have tried to sketch briefly the rationales that are given by two important constituencies, and a brief sample of other views from around the world. In practical terms, it will probably be far more fruitful for us now to collaborate in seeking ways to lessen the risks of excessive drinking and the harms that result from it.... There may be other words that convey similar meanings adequately, without the problematic use of the term "alcohol and other drugs" (CSAP/ICAP Joint Working Group on Terminology 1998).

Public-health advocates criticized the CSAP, which in the mid-1990s almost lost its federal budget as a result of heavy alcohol industry lobbying of Congress, for participating in issuing a report that obfuscates the scientific fact that alcohol is a drug. Some interpreted CSAP's action as caving in to Big Alcohol. ICAP also issued a policy statement recommending that governments should join with the alcohol industry and private foundations in researching the relationship between drinking, pleasure, and good health (Abramson 1998).

Critical to CSAP's approach, indeed that of the entire alcohol industry was the erection of a conceptual and cultural barrier between alcohol and other, especially, illicit drugs. The objective was to portray alcohol as a necessary, normal, and valuable part of everyday life, and hence not really a drug at all. Public policies followed accordingly, with alcohol being treated as a somewhat controlled consumable commodity and illicit drugs being rendered as the real psychotropic threats to society. Public health statistics showing that alcohol consumption does far more harm to society than all forms of illicit drug consumption combined, underline the considerable social distance between the worlds of drug research and the worlds of policy formulation about drugs.

BANNING MARIHUANA

Despite Prohibition's ultimate failure, the US government, as well as the governments of states and local municipalities, repeatedly enacted laws that had the same intention: to forbid people from consuming drugs said to be harmful to the consumers. Among the measures taken by these governments were the 1937 Federal Marihuana Tax Act; various state and local laws against possession, transport, or sale of marihuana; state and local laws against possession of paraphernalia for consuming drugs; and more recently, draconian laws against possession, transport, or sale of crack cocaine. The development of the legal system that now comprises the drug-control regime in the United States did not come into being as whole cloth, but rather in pieces large and small, local, state, and federal, with a focus often on specific drugs rather than the panoply of available psychoactive drugs. An early and enduring target was marihuana.

During the colonial era, marihuana or hemp was a cash crop grown to provide material used in the production of both clothing and rope, and it is still grown for these purposes. By the turn of the 20th century, marihuana was being sold as an over-the-counter medicine for the relief of various minor aches and ailments. It appeared primarily as an ingredient in corn plasters, in nonintoxicating medicaments, and as a component in several veterinary medicines. Its status for medicinal purposes was affirmed in the Pure Food and Drug Act of 1906, which required that any quantity of marihuana be clearly indicated on the labels of products sold to the public.

Then, during the 1920s, marihuana began to be used in the United States as a recreational drug for its mood- and mind-altering effects. This phase began with the transport of increasing quantities of marihuana from Mexico and the Caribbean into the United States after the First World War. As the popularity of marihuana grew, a significant social reaction occurred. The drug soon was labeled a dangerous narcotic and attempts were made to institute severe penalties for its use.

Attempts to criminalize marihuana use did not go unopposed. During 1911 hearings on a federal antinarcotic law by the House Ways and Means Committee, for example, the National Wholesale Druggists' Association protested the inclusion of marihuana as a dangerous drug. Efforts by the pharmaceutical industry to block federal legislation outlawing the sale of marihuana were successful until 1937, when the Marijuana Tax Act was passed. This legislation was directly linked to an effort to stop the flow of Mexican workers into the American Southwest. While these workers had been welcomed in the 1920s to fill the demand for farm labor, during the Great Depression of the 1930s they came to be seen as an unwelcome labor surplus. Nationalistic anti-Mexican immigration groups (not terribly different than those we see today) began to form with the objective of painting marihuana as an insidious narcotic used and distributed by an unwanted group of foreign residents who needed to be deported. As the editor of the Alamosa, Colorado, *Daily Courier* expressed this unabashedly racist sentiment in an editorial published in 1936: "I wish I could show you what a small marihuana cigarette can do to one of our degenerate Spanish-speaking residents. That's why our problem is so great: the greatest percentage of our population is composed of Spanish-speaking persons, most of whom are low mentally" (reprinted in Musto 1987:223). This chauvinistic campaign to block Mexican immigration contributed to the marihuana scare of the 1930s and to the federal inclusion of marihuana as a narcotic despite its clear chemical differences from narcotizing drugs.

This process was aided and abetted by Harry Anslinger, a former railroad policeman and outgoing assistant commissioner of the US Bureau of Prohibition, who in 1930 was appointed as the first commissioner to the newly created Federal Bureau of Narcotics (FBN). In this role, Anslinger became convinced that there was an alarming rise in the use of marihuana occurring in the country. In response, he initiated an effort to convince Congress to pass legislation that would place the distribution of marihuana under the control of the FBN. As part of this effort, he launched a radio campaign against marihuana and took his anti-marihuana message on the road to his various speaking engagements. In effect, in 1936 Anslinger "declared war on marihuana" (Carroll 2004:70).

This development is noteworthy because until this point he had largely ignored the drug, because he did not see it as addictive or in the same category of threat as opium or cocaine. His about face has been interpreted as a political move to forestall the disintegration of his job as part of the Secret Service Reorganization Act that was then being supported by President Roosevelt to increase federal-government efficiency. Marihuana, presented to the public as a looming danger of untold proportions, provided a target that justified retaining his office (Carroll 2004). In his first radio address on the topic, Anslinger (1937) adopted the dramatic language of moral panic to drive home his message:

> The habit appears to be gaining ground rapidly. The gravity of this menace, the pernicious effects of the use of marihuana, and the necessity for eradication, should be brought forcibly before the notice of our people.

Thus began a strategy of painting marihuana as a demonic substance linked to violent crime, loss of control of will power, and complete destruction of sexual inhibition, themes that Anslinger promoted and others readily adopted in what became a mounting crusade to re-invent marihuana in socially useful if factually unjustifiable ways. Along the way, as the campaign heated up, the Secret Service Reorganization Act failed to pass Congress and faded from Washington's volatile political stage. Anslinger emerged on the national scene as a law-and-order drug evangelist who embraced the most extreme and violent stereotypes of marihuana users. In his testimony before Congress in 1937 in support of the Marihuana Tax Act, he stated that after using marihuana

> Some individuals have a complete loss of sense of time or a sense of value. They lose their sense of place. [They] have an increased feeling of physical strength and power. Some people will fly into a delirious rage, and they are temporarily irresponsible and may commit violent crimes.... It is dangerous to the mind and body, and particularly dangerous to the criminal type, because it releases all of the inhibitions.... There was one town in Ohio where a young man went into a hotel and held up the clerk and killed him, and his defense was that he had been affected by the use of marihuana.... In Florida a 21-year-old boy under the influence of this drug killed his parents and his brothers and sisters. The evidence showed that he had smoked marihuana. In Chicago recently two boys murdered a policeman while under the influence of marihuana. Not long ago we found a 15-year-old boy going insane because, the doctor told the enforcement officers, he thought the boy was smoking marihuana cigarettes (Anslinger 1937).

As part of the anti-marihuana campaign, a high level Conference on *Cannabis sativa* was convened in Washington, DC in January of 1937. Conferees included doctors, researchers, lawyers, and government officials like Anslinger. Following this meeting, a barrage of marihuana horror stories were printed in the media, including an article that Anslinger co-authored with Courtney Ryley Cooper (1937) titled "Marijuana: Assassin of Youth," that appeared in *American Magazine*. Other articles with similar sensationalistic titles like "Youth Gone Loco," "One More Peril for Youth," "Marijuana—A New Menace to U.S.," "Uncle Sam Fights New Drug Menace—Marihuana," and "Marihuana: Increasing Use and Terrifying Effects" began showing up in magazines like the *American Mercury, Scientific American, Popular Science Monthly, Christian Century, Survey Graphic,* and *Literary Digest* during the late 1930s. The media frenzy helped to create a national climate that secured passage of the Marijuana Tax Act.

Following passage of the Act, popular use of the drug and general social concern about marihuana began to flag. Penalties for marihuana use were increased periodically, but its use stabilized among certain social sectors. For the most part, marihuana disappeared from the front pages of newspapers and from other forums of public discussion. All of this changed again with the sudden reemergence of marihuana in the 1960s. At this point, marihuana led a wave of new youth-centered drug use that continues to have impact 50 years later.

Researchers have had a difficult time understanding and classifying the effects of marihuana or of delta-nine tetrahydrocannabinol, its primary psychoactive component. Effects appear to vary based on the local setting and set of cultural expectations (cf. Zinberg and Weil 1969). Working-class Jamaicans, for example, among whom use is widespread, do not expect hallucinogenic reactions to ganja, as marihuana is known on the island. Therefore, reports of c annabis-induced hallucinations are not regularly reported among Jamaican ganja smokers. Rather, in Jamaica marihuana use is linked culturally with values of endurance, energy, problem solving, invigoration of appetite, and relaxation. As the anthropologists Vera Rubin and Lambros Comitas (1983:214) indicate,

> Ganja use is integrally linked to all aspects of working-class social structure; cultivation, cash crops, marketing, and economics; consumer-cultivator-dealer networks; intraclass relationships and processes of avoidance and cooperation; parent-child, peer, and mate relationships; folk medicine; folk religious doctrines; obeah and gossip sanctions; personality and culture; interclass stereotypes; legal and church sanctions; perceived requisites of behavioral changes for social mobility; and adaptive strategies.

Among participants in the ganja subculture, affording and acquiring the drug, anticipating the next use, efforts to avoid detection by the police, and the sense of community among fellow users all contribute to the importance of ganja at the individual and small-group levels. Moreover, regular users strongly dispute allegations that use leads to crime, violence, apathy, physical and mental health problems, or an antisocial attitude. Based on their field study in Jamaica, Rubin and Comitas (1983:217) concluded, "There is no evidence of any causal relationship between cannabis use and mental deterioration, insanity, violence or poverty; or that widespread cannabis use in Jamaica produces an apathetic, indolent class of people."

This kind of finding populates the academic drug literature, often to the disgruntlement of government funders of marihuana research. The federal classification of cannabis and its organic compounds as Schedule I prohibited drugs (a designation reserved for the most inebriating drugs that are seen as having no medical value) is seen by many drug researchers as scientifically unsupportable, as expressed in a government-sponsored review of the literature published in *The Open Neurology Journal* (Grant et al. 2012). Investigators at the University of California at San Diego and the University of California, Davis, reviewed the results of several recent clinical trials assessing the safety and efficacy of inhaled or vaporized cannabis and concluded that "Based on evidence currently available the Schedule I classification is not tenable; it is not accurate that cannabis has no medical value, or that information on safety is lacking" (Grant et al. 2012). As this statement suggests, key elements of US drug policy are neither based on nor informed by empirical research.

Available research notwithstanding, the criminalization of marihuana use and the extensive incarceration of those caught with even small amounts of marihuana remains in full force—constituting what many have come to view as a real incarnation of "reefer madness"—although challenges of various sorts, from a push for legalization for medicinal purposes (such as the 1996 passage of legislation in both California and Arizona, and the passage thus far of similar legislation in 17 states and Washington, DC) or the passage of state laws and referendums decriminalizing possession of small quantities of marihuana (as occurred in two states, Colorado and Washington, in the 2012 national elections), are growing.

The response of the federal government during the Obama administration to the legalization movement has been consistent opposition to any form of legalization and a repeated commitment to the enforcement of the Controlled Substances Act. As the Office of National Drug Control Policy (2012) reiterated on its webpage

- Marijuana use is associated with dependence, respiratory and mental illness, poor motor performance, and impaired cognitive and immune system functioning, among other negative effects.
- Marijuana intoxication can cause distorted perceptions, difficulty in thinking and problem solving, and problems with learning and memory.
- Studies have shown an association between chronic marihuana use and increased rates of anxiety, depression, suicidal thoughts, and schizophrenia.
- Marijuana smoke contains carcinogens and is an irritant to the lungs. Marijuana smoke, in fact, contains 50–70 percent more carcinogenic hydrocarbons than does tobacco smoke.

Consequently, the US Department of Justice is likely to file lawsuits challenging efforts to legalize marihuana in Colorado and Washington.

One significant product of this view of marihuana as a looming threat is that incarceration rates have dramatically increased even though crime rates have remained stable or even declined (Smith 2004). What has gone up, however, is arrest rates for marihuana violations. In 2009, for example, according to the Federal Bureau of Investigation's annual Uniform Crime Report, police around the country prosecuted 858,408 persons for marihuana violations, a 1.3 percent increase in the number of such arrests reported for the prior year (Armentano 2010). According to the report, marihuana arrests now comprise over half (approximately 52 percent) of all drug arrests reported in the United States. A decade ago, by contrast, arrests for marihuana violations comprised only 44 percent of all drug arrests. Moreover, of those individuals charged with marihuana violations, approximately 88 percent were charged only with possession, not with the sale or manufacture of the drug.

How are we to understand the explosive increase in the arrest and incarceration of people for the possession of marihuana since the mid-1970s? According to Smith's (2004:925) analysis,

> [R]ather than crime or a structural response to citizen attitudes, incarceration rates have increased because of Republican electoral successes at the state level, the nature of executive elections, and the continuing legacy of a racial social rift. It is politics in their most basic form, and in particular specific and identifiable state-level policies and political processes that explain why incarceration rates in the 1980s and 1990s became increasingly disconnected from crime rates.

Lubricating this political process has been the aggressive public demonization of the marihuana user. For the Drug Enforcement Administration (DEA), this has meant continued stress on the image of the marihuana user as a criminal, apt to be involved in various nefarious activities. As noted in The DEA Position on Marijuana (DEA 2011) posted on the DEA website,

> Marijuana is known to contribute to delinquent and aggressive *behavior....* Moreover, early use of marijuana, the most commonly used drug among teens, is a warning sign for later criminal behavior. Specifically, research shows that the instances of physically attacking people, stealing property, and destroying property increase in direct proportion to the frequency with which teens smoke marijuana.

In other words, research be damned, what is *still* needed is a strict law-and-order approach that emphasizes an orientation that favors getting tough on crime and no coddling drug criminals, as the latter are threats to society that can only be controlled through long and painful incarceration.

THE EVIL COUPLE: HEROIN AND COCAINE

While marihuana is the most widely used illicit drug, the two most significant hard drugs throughout US history have been cocaine and the opiates (including heroin). Both of these in their various forms have a long and colorful history of use. Cocaine, derived from the leaves of the coca plant (*Erythroxlon coca*), has long been chewed among the Indians of the Andes as a mild stimulant that has various positive effects at high altitudes and produces no health or social consequences. The Spanish invaders at first attempted to eliminate the chewing of coca leaves, in part because of its pagan religious connections, and because they perceived coca chewing as unsightly and unsanitary, rather than because of an antidrug sentiment. When they discovered, however, that coca use facilitated the hard labor performed by indigenous people in Spanish mines, they began to distribute it to workers daily. Western interest in drugs like cocaine began with the discovery of quinine as a treatment for malarial fever. That a substance derived from a plant could be used with great effect in the treatment of a specific health problem generated an intense curiosity about discovering other new plant-based medicinals. This drive led to the identification and refinement of the psychotropically active ingredient in coca and its production and use in an array of legal consumer products including wines, soft drinks, and so-called patent medicines (none of which actually held a government patent).

Social valuing of cocaine, however, ran head on into attitudes about cocaine (as well as heroin and other opiates) colored by racist prejudice. Throughout the American South, for example, there developed a fear that if blacks had access to cocaine they "might become oblivious of their prescribed bounds and attack white society" (Musto 1987:6). Thus, in 1903, the *New York Tribune* quoted Colonel J. W. Watson of Georgia asserting "many of the horrible crimes committed in the Southern States by colored people can be traced directly to the cocaine habit" (quoted in Goode 1984:186). Similarly, the *New York Times* published an article entitled "Negro Cocaine Fiends Are a New Southern Menace" that described blacks as "running amuck in a cocaine frenzy" (quoted in Goode 1984:186). That African Americans were on the receiving end of most of the racially motivated horrible crimes committed in the South during this period was of little consequence, as facts rarely get in the way of strong or useful belief. As Musto (1987:7) notes,

The fear of the cocainized black coincided with the peak of lynchings, legal segregation, and voting laws all designed to remove political and social power from [blacks].... One of the most terrifying beliefs about cocaine was that it actually improved pistol marksmanship. Another myth, that cocaine made blacks almost unaffected by mere .32 caliber bullets, is said to have caused southern police departments to switch to .38 caliber revolvers. These fantasies characterized white fear, not the reality of cocaine's effects, and gave one more reason for the repression of blacks.

Ironically, these politically motivated fears were not only misguided with respect to cocaine's effects, they were motivated by erroneous ideas about African American access to cocaine. In fact, the cost of the drug (twenty-five cents per grain in 1910) prohibited most African Americans in the South, the majority of whom were sharecroppers and conspicuously poorer on average than whites, from purchasing the drug during this period. A study by E. M. Green (1914), who examined admissions to Georgia State Sanitarium at the time, showed that rates of cocaine use by blacks in the South were significantly lower than rates of white use. Nonetheless, to insure that cocaine in any form did not reach African Americans, it was dropped as an ingredient in Coca-Cola in 1903 and replaced by another stimulant, caffeine. Also that year, the British Committee on the Acquirement of Drug Habits described cocaine users as typically "bohemians, gamblers, high- and low-class prostitutes, night porters, bell boys, burglars, racketeers, pimps, and casual laborers" (quoted in Feiling 2010). Reflecting this social trend, the Pure Food and Drug Act required the listing of cocaine as an active ingredient in consumer goods beginning in 1906.

In short order, the federal Harrison Narcotics Tax Act passed in 1914, leading to the eventual (but far from immediate) outlawing of the sale and distribution of cocaine in the United States. In an effort to secure tax revenue from the importation and sale of cocaine, and reduce the number of the American populace that were addicted to opium, those supporting passage of the Harrison Act, like Representative Francis Burton Harrison of New York who proposed it, appealed to the fears of "drug-crazed, sex-mad negroes" and made references to Negroes under the influence of drugs murdering whites, degenerate Mexicans smoking marihuana, and "Chinamen" seducing white women with drugs. In providing testimony in support of passage of the Harrison Act, Christopher Koch of Pennsylvania's State Pharmacy Board made often repeated racial innuendos about blacks and cocaine explicit when he stated that, "Most of the attacks upon the white women of the South are the direct result of a cocaine-crazed Negro brain" (quoted in Feiling 2010). Similarly, Dr. Hamilton Wright testified that drugs made blacks uncontrollable, gave African Americans superhuman powers and caused them to rebel against white authority.

Yet cocaine was not considered a controlled substance until 1970, when the US government listed it as such in the Comprehensive Drug Abuse Prevention and Control Act. Until that point, the use of cocaine was only rarely prosecuted in the United States. The shift in attitudes about cocaine constituted the long brewing development of a moral panic in an anxious social body conflicted about its attitudes about drugs but ever fearful of the angered rise of subordinated and potentially vengeful social groups known to be the victims of exploitive abuse.

The other long-standing hard drug in use in the America pharmacopeia, opium "was one of the products Columbus hoped to bring back" from his voyages to his benefactors, the royalty of Spain (Scott 1969:11). While opium was not to be found in the New World that Columbus stumbled upon on his way to Asia, the drug would eventually be imported to meet a growing demand. When the use of opiates actually began in what became the United States is not entirely clear, but it is known to have been sometime during the colonial period. Critical to its introduction was the work of one of the best-known British doctors of the 17th century, a man named Thomas Sydenham. A founder of clinical medicine, Sydenham advocated the use of opium as "one of the most valued medicines in the world [which] does more honor to medicine than any remedy whatsoever" (quoted in Musto 1987:69). In his view, without opium, "the healing arts would cease to exist" (Scott 1969:114).

During the 1800s, opium use was widespread in the United States; it was treated as a normal behavior that was both legal and integrated into everyday activities. People of all walks of life became addicted, especially a large number of urban middle-class housewives who were often the targets of the first generation of media advertising efforts. Addiction, however, was usually not recognized as such, since the drug was readily available and widely used (and those who were addicted could easily treat their withdrawal symptoms through continued drug consumption). Thus, regular use of opium in powder or tincture form was not defined socially as a significant problem. Users were not labeled criminals or deviants, although heavy use certainly was frowned on and behaviors now associated with addiction did carry a certain level of social disapproval.

By contrast, a behavior that was labeled as a drug problem was the smoking of opium in opium dens, primarily run, as we have seen in literary references discussed in Chapter 4, by Chinese immigrants (who were brought to the United States to do the hard labor of laying railroad rails, digging mines, and building levees). The first anti-opium law in the nation was passed locally in San Francisco in 1875, home to a large Chinese population. Smoking was labeled deviant and debilitating, but the real problem appears to have been racism. The primary concern was not drug use per se but who was using the drugs. This interpretation is supported by a temporally related case tried in Oregon and reviewed in an Oregon district court. The defendant in the case was a Chinese man convicted of selling opium. In the review, the district court noted: "Smoking opium is not our vice, and therefore, it may be that this legislation proceeds more from a desire to vex and annoy the 'Heathen Chinese' in this respect, than to protect the people from the evil habit" (quoted in Bonnie and Whitebread 1970:997).

From this moment forward, US societal reaction to drug use and negative attitudes about particular ethnic groups have been closely intertwined. In the case of Chinese opium smoking, an essential factor in social condemnation was the depression that began in the 1860s and the resulting redefinition of the Chinese as surplus labor. Originally, imported to perform labor that was unappealing to many US workers, the Chinese later became scapegoats of class frustration as the economy collapsed. Lines were drawn, distinctions made, particular behaviors embellished or invented, and harshly judged, resulting in the Chinese being defined as existing outside the social boundaries of American society (followed shortly by efforts to drive them beyond the geographic borders of the nation). This example reveals an important aspect of US experience with illicit drugs that is often hidden behind well-publicized events like so-called wars on drugs or media hype about crack babies. As Helmer (1983:27) has argued, "the conflict over social justice is what the story of narcotics in America is about."

The place of opium use in American society took a dramatic turn in 1803 with the discovery of the means of making morphine water soluable. Ten times more potent than raw opium, morphine was quickly realized to have tremendous powers as a painkiller; morphine, in fact, remains the strongest chemical pain reliever available. This fact became significant during the American Civil War, an enormously bloody conflict that threatened to overwhelm the capacity of the mid-19th century medical system. Physicians turned eagerly to morphine as a means of handling the incredible number of war-inflicted wounds and amputations they faced. This process was facilitated by the invention of the hypodermic needle, which allowed the rapid introduction of the drug to areas of pain within the body. One product of widespread morphine use during and after the Civil War was the emergence of a new medical condition called either "soldier's disease" or "army disease." Its primary symptom was morphine craving by those who had been medically treated with the drug. The treatment adopted by physicians was to continue morphine injections for those who presented with this disease.

Passage of the Harrison Act also had a big impact, of an increasing nature on opium users. But legal moves against this drug by the federal government actually began in the international arena. In 1909 and 1911, the United States convened an international opium conference, which produced a document called the Hague Convention of 1912, aimed at restricting international traffic in opium. Under the leadership of William Jennings Bryan, Congress followed up with provisions in the Harrison Act that placed restrictions on the sale of over-the-counter opium preparations. Congressional debate about passage of these measures did not center on the negative health effects of opium or the threat of the opium user to society, nor even on the rising rate of addiction in the US population, but rather on issues of international relations and profit. In particular, the discussion focused on the fact that the British were gaining an economic windfall from their ability to press opium sales on China and thereby achieve a competitive edge against US businesses globally.

The ultimate social effect of the new federal anti-drug law, however, was the labeling of the drug user as undesirable and criminal. In the aftermath of this moral cataloguing, drug use came to be synonymous with deviance, lack of control, violence, and social decay. By the 1920s, "the public image of the addict had become that of a criminal, a willful degenerate, a hedonistic thrill-seeker in need of imprisonment and stiff punishment" (Goode 1984:218).

Physicians were exempt from the Harrison Act, and they continued to treat their addicted patients with opium (as well as cocaine); as a result, thousands of people continued legal drug use in this way for five years after passage of the Harrison Act. In the aftermath of the Harrison Act, physicians set up clinics around the country to dispense mind-altering drugs to addicted patients. In the New York clinic, which was the one best known to the public, drugs were handed out widely to those who claimed addiction. Some people eventually began to take their dose plus additional doses for resale on the street to other newly recruited addicts. Thus began the underground narcotics industry.

Before long the US Treasury Department, which was assigned to enforce the Harrison Act, began to press against the legal prescription of psychoactive drugs even by doctors. Central to this drive was the growing concern, energized by a kind of trickle-up theory, that drug use would spread from the working class "into the higher social ranks of the country" (Helmer 1983:16). In 1919, in the Supreme Court case of Webb versus the United States, it was decided that a physician could not prescribe a narcotic to an addict simply to avoid the pain of withdrawal. In 1922, in a second Supreme Court case, the United States versus Behrman, the court ruled that narcotics could not be prescribed even as part of a cure. The effect was to make it now impossible for addicts to gain legal access to drugs: "The clinics shut their doors and a new figure appeared on the American scene—the pusher" (McCoy et al. 1986:110).

At first, physicians resisted these new legal developments. In the 12 years after passage of the Harrison Act, at least 25,000 physicians were arrested on narcotics-selling charges, and 3,000 served time in jail as a result. Thousands more had their licenses revoked. By 1923, all of the drug clinics, even those that had been fairly successful in weaning addicts off drugs, were shut down. By 1919, there were 1,000 addicts brought up on federal drug charges. By 1925, there were 10,000 arrests per year. The end result of these developments was the emergence and continued existence of an underground drug subculture that functioned to enable addicts to gain access to drugs and drug injection equipment and to avoid arrest. Ultimately, this population was targeted by the War on Drugs.

THE LONGEST WAR

The United States war in Vietnam lasted from 1956 (the date of the first US casualty) until 1975, and thus has gained the designation as being the longest war in US history. Although a different kind of war, the War on Drug began (officially) with President Richard Nixon's declaration in 1971. Nevertheless, the policies that his administration implemented as part of the Comprehensive Drug Abuse Prevention and Control Act were a continuation and enhancement of drug-prohibition policies dating to the Harrison Act. Thus the War on Drugs (terminology officially dropped by the Obama administration, without much other change in actual practice) is truly, and by far, the oldest war in US history.

Particularly since the Korean War, there has been a consistent and growing federal effort to implement new policies and programs designed to stop the use of some drugs. These efforts significantly intensified in response to the radical increase in drug use that occurred, especially among youth and young adults, beginning in the mid-1960s. As Musto (1987:253) comments,

"The use of illegal drugs increased astoundingly in the 1960s. Drugs thought safely interred with the past, marihuana and heroin, rapidly resurfaced at the same time that new drugs such as LSD materialized and attained tremendous popularity." Ultimately, the movement of drugs onto primarily white college campuses and among other white middle-class youth culminated in Richard Nixon labeling drugs "public enemy number one" (use among youth of color dating to the post–Second World War period never roused such concern).

War or no war, it is apparent that once it is established drug supply-and-demand chains are not easy to eradicate, although patterns change over time as do user populations. As journalist, magazine editor, and political commentator H. L. Mencken (1917) wrote, "There is always an easy solution to every human problem—neat, plausible, and wrong." He might have been talking about the War on Drugs. Thus, as Nadelmann (2007:1) observes, "global production and consumption of drugs are roughly the same as they were a decade ago; meanwhile, many producers have become more efficient, and cocaine and heroin have become purer and cheaper." This point, he elaborates (Nadelman 2007) by asserting,

> Looking to the United States as a role model for drug control is like looking to apartheid-era South Africa for how to deal with race.... And yet, despite [its] dismal record [in the War on Drugs], the United States has succeeded in constructing an international drug-prohibition regime modeled after its own highly punitive and moralistic approach. It has dominated the drug-control agencies of the United Nations and other international organizations, and its federal drug-enforcement agency was the first national police organization to go global. Rarely has one nation so successfully promoted its own failed policies to the rest of the world.

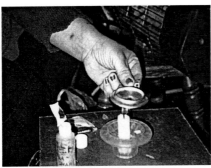

Drug use preparation in Denver (Photo by Robert Booth)

Over the last 40 years, the price tag for US War on Drugs has been in the neighborhood $1 trillion and hundreds of thousands of lives. Every 20 seconds, someone in the United States is arrested for a drug violation, and at the rate of one per week, a new prison is erected to house the unprecedented throng of inmates that are kept behind bars in the world's largest and most populated penal system (Singer 2004). In New York State, for example, the Rockefeller Drug Laws of 1973 radically restricted judicial discretion in utilizing alternatives to incarceration as a response to drug offenses. The result of the enactment of these laws was that while 11 percent of the total state prison population in 1980 were individuals incarcerated for drug-related offenses by January of 2008, that figure was 33 percent (Correction Association of New York 2011). Although it has only 5 percent of the world's population, 25 percent of the world's prison population is behind bars in US jails and prisons. Further, more African Americans today are under criminal justice supervision—either in prison, on parole or probation—than were enslaved 10 years before the Civil War (Alexander 2012). Additionally, more than 10 percent of black men between 20 and 35 years of age are incarcerated, which separates them from their families and children. The War on Drugs, in short, has been experienced in minority communities as a savage War on People. As Klieman and colleagues (2012) conclude, "The U.S. has reached a dead end in trying to fight drug use by treating every offender as a serious criminal."

POLICIES, LAWS, AND PRACTICES THAT ADD VALUE TO THE USELESS

Revelations over the years have shown that government and international efforts to control drugs often are colored by political motives that have little to do with curbing the harmful effects drugs might have. Indeed, one common argument about why such a failed war and the failed policies it reflects continue is that it reaps a set of secondary gains for those who promote it (Blackman 2010). Such gains involve the use of the useless by others with a political, economic, or alternative self-interest in the Othering and control of drug users.

The starting point for amplified efforts to put drug users to use lies in a deeply engrained perception of drug users even among those who have never met one in their lives, although they certainly have encountered them by way of the books, movies, news reports, or other venues discussed in previous chapters. Noted Peretti-Watel (2003:321),

> [T]he stereotype of the "dopefiend" seems useless, since heroin users remain unfamiliar to most people. Nevertheless, conceiving a perfect stranger as a devil who concentrates all the vices (the "dope fiend" is supposed to steal, to lie or even to kill, without being able to control himself ...) can prove useful in order to reassure our values, to draw a

clear boundary between good and evil: our moral universe is inhabited by many stereotypes which are clearly either good or bad, and which provide us with models to follow as well as with scarecrows to avoid.

Not only are drug users good to moralize with, always available to hold up as negative role models and hapless scape goats, they have other, often hidden, values as well, that are covered over and made possible by the War on Drugs. In addition, as Chambliss (1994) argued, the War on Drugs has "produced another war as well: it is the war between the police and minority youth." African Americans, who comprise about 12 percent of the US population, make up 55 percent of those convicted on drug charges. Rarely addressed in the War on Drugs is any systematic assessment of why socially marginalized working-class youth turn to drug use or involvement in the drug trade (mostly at lower levels of street distribution). The answer, however, appears to be that the illicit drug trade is "the biggest equal opportunity employer" (Bourgois 2003b:320) for inner city youth, males and females alike.

Fourth, by creating an exploitable pariah group of low-cost drug-dependent workers, and by allowing the development of a revolving system for warehousing segments of the labor force behind prison bars, the War on Drugs lowers production costs and increases corporate profits. As Alisse Waterston (1993:241) pointed out, "As a special category, addicts are politically weak and disconnected from organized labor, thereby becoming a source of cheap, easily expendable labor." The existence of this group drags down wages for everyone, because each layer of the labor force enables employers to lower the wages paid to layers above it (because cheaper workers are portrayed as ready and willing to take their jobs for lower wages and fewer benefits). Prisoners arrested on drug charges wind up as part of an incarcerated labor pool for private corporations (e.g., in assembly) for very low wages and society, rather than the employer, pays the cost of sustaining this work force (e.g., food, clothes, medical care, shelter). Further, as Chien and colleagues (2000:19) indicate, employers of prisoners "can freely dismiss and recall workers [and] need not deal with unions."

Fifth, beginning in the mid-1980s, the United States began to outsource prison construction and operation. The first private prison contract was awarded in 1984 to Corrections Corporation of America (CCA), which remains the largest for-profit prison company in the country. Seeking locations that would not reject the presence of a prison, private prisons often selected communities hard hit by corporate flight and the globalized economy. Heavily subsidized by taxpayer money even before receiving public contracts, private companies were able to build prisons throughout the country. For every convicted individual sent to one of its prisons, the CCA or other private prison operator receives approximately $122 a day. Based on this revenue flow, the CCA reported $1.7 billion in gross income in 2011, about half from government contracts (Carlsen 2012). But this was a time of falling crime rates. The real challenge for private prisons became filling all the cells in their newly erected prisons with convicted offenders. To drum up business, the private prison industry turned to lobbying in order to win stiff drug and immigration policies. The CCA 2010 Annual Report straightforwardly lays out the need for criminalization by warning its investors:

> The demand for our facilities could be adversely affected by the relaxation of enforcement efforts, leniency in conviction or parole standards and sentencing practices or through the decriminalization of certain activities that are currently proscribed by our criminal laws. For instance, any changes with respect to drugs and controlled substances or illegal immigration could affect the number of persons arrested, convicted and sentenced, thereby potentially reducing demand for correctional facilities to house them (quoted in Riggs 2012).

To insure a steady stream of new prisoners, while doing little if anything to boost public safety, private prison companies over the last decade spent over $45 million lobbying law makers. Whenever new bills that increased police power to detain suspected criminals, criminalize behaviors (such as adding new drugs to those that are illegal to sell or use) or extending prison sentences, private prisons could be found making significant campaign contributions to office holders. For example, lobbyists for the private prison industry have pushed for passage of "three strikes" and "truth-in-sentencing" laws across the country. Both of these types of laws adversely impact drug users. Some of the tactics employed by private prison companies, or individuals affiliated with them, to gain influence or acquire new contracts or inmates flows included: "the use of questionable financial incentives; benefitting from the "revolving door" between public and private corrections; extensive lobbying; lavish campaign contributions; and efforts to control information" (ACLU 2011). As a result of such labors, as the ACLU (2011) points out, "the crippling cost of imprisoning increasing numbers of Americans saddles government budgets with rising debt and exacerbates the current fiscal crises confronting states across the nation."

A set of citizens that are readily amenable to mobilization in support of campaigns for new laws or new prisons are prison employees. Prison-guard unions have a strong vested interest in keeping people incarcerated in high numbers. In 2008, the California Correctional Peace Officers Association, for example, spent $1 million to defeat a measure that would have reduced sentences and parole times for nonviolent drug offenders while emphasizing drug treatment over imprisonment (Fang 2012). Additionally, police departments throughout the country have become dependent on federal drug war grants to finance their budgets. To keep this money flowing, police unions see it in their best interests to lobby against drug legalization. For example, the successful campaign in 2010 against Proposition 19 in California, a ballot measure to legalize marihuana, was coordinated by a police-union lobbyist. These efforts helped insure that the police department would collect tens of millions in federal marihuana-eradication grants. Federal lobbying disclosures reveal that other police-union lobbyists around the country also pushed for stiffer penalties for marihuana-related crimes.

Sixth, civil-asset-forfeiture laws have been passed that empower the seizures of private property even without charging anyone with violation of a law, and hence without having to prove illegal behavior beyond a reasonable doubt. Seized property, such as fast boats used to smuggle illegal drugs, is presumed to be illicitly gained or used, and can be confiscated by a police department or other government body based solely on hearsay evidence, such as a tip supplied by a government informant who stands to gain up to 25 percent of the forfeited assets. Confiscation may occur without an arrest because it is defined legally as an arrest of property, rather than an arrest of a person, and the necessity of proving a party guilty is not required. Numerous police, sheriff, and related law-enforcement departments around the country have embraced forfeiture laws to boost their departmental budgets significantly, and their various budget-related perks. A study involving 90 interviews with law-enforcement officials, prosecutors, and forfeiture attorneys around the nation (Burnett 2008) suggested that police agencies that reported they were seizing property or drug money to help finance the War on Drugs appeared to be mainly doing so to help increase their own departmental budgets. Also, existing evidence shows that some officers use their badges to take cash from drivers stopped on the road for alleged drug-related suspicions without any evidence. Researchers have identified numerous examples of questionable purchases made with seized money or from money made by selling off seized assets, including:

- Albany, New York, Police Department: Was found to have spent $7,711 from confiscations on photographs of police officers and artwork for administrative offices, and $16,190 on food, gifts, and entertainment.

- Colorado State Patrol: Was found to have paid from confiscated funds $832 for knives as incentive awards; $599 on embroidered polo shirts; $907 for tickets to minor-league baseball games; $1,410 for fleece vests and bomber jackets; $107 for poker chips; $234 at Bath & Body Works for various items.
- St. Louis County Police Department: Used confiscation money in the amount of $144,689 to reimburse employees for courses taken at local colleges and universities to complete bachelor's or master's degree programs, such as English Composition, Advanced Contract Law, and Introduction to Astronomy.
- Fulton County, Georgia, District Attorney's Office: Paid $5,000 in forfeited money for an annual Christmas party, including a red cape printed with "Super Lawyer," $6,650 on dinners, college football tickets, fundraisers, and galas.
- Boston Police Department: Spent $2.6 million in confiscation funds to lease SUVs, sedans, and other vehicles for eight years. The Department says the vehicles were assigned to undercover officers trying to fit into drug scenes.

As these examples suggest, confiscation laws have turned the War on Drugs into a plentiful font of easily gained funds, allowing, in some cases, for law enforcement offices to be completely financed through seized property and cash, primarily from alleged drug dealers (many of whom were never brought to trial). We cite just a few examples, but given the pervasiveness of drug consumption and the traffic that serves it, we can safely assume that many more police departments and sheriff's offices have availed themselves of the "system's" advantages. One result of these windfalls has been a collapse of public oversight of police because taxpayers have afforded decreasing support for law enforcement. The windfalls from confiscation laws gained the War on Drugs a large cadre of law-enforcement supporters who benefited from seized assets, both legally and through local corruption. Concluded Blumenson and Nilsen (1998), forfeiture laws and practices and other components of the War on Drugs have undermined rather than enhanced law enforcement:

> During the past decade, law enforcement agencies increasingly have turned to asset seizures and drug enforcement grants to compensate for budgetary shortfalls, at the expense of other criminal justice goals. We believe the strange shape of the criminal justice system today—the law enforcement agenda that targets assets rather than crime . . . the 80

percent of seizures that are unaccompanied by any criminal prosecution … the plea bargains that favor drug kingpins and penalize the "mules" without assets to trade … the reverse stings that target drug buyers rather than drug sellers … the overkill in agencies involved even in minor arrests … the massive shift towards federal jurisdiction over local law enforcement … —is largely the unplanned by-product of this economic incentive structure.

THE PERSONAL IMPACT OF POLICY— EFFECTS ON THE LIVES OF DRUG USERS

The effects of stringent drug laws on the people who use prohibited drugs often seem to exacerbate the effects of the drug use in unintended ways. For example, the crackdown on script doctors (those physicians who readily write psychotropic drug prescriptions for their patients) and possession of injection paraphernalia were intended to prevent people from self-injecting opioids. In fact, opioid users found street-based sources for their drug of choice, but had to inject it intravenously to get the desired effect. Intravenous injection led to contamination of the needle and syringe with often infectious blood, and because access to injection equipment was limited, the users adapted by re-using already contaminated equipment previously put to use by other people. These processes led to risks associated with self-injection, including local abscesses (due to use of well-worn and dull needles), hepatitis B, hepatitis C syphilis, and HIV infection. Causal sequences like this one abound in the experience of drug ethnographers but do not dissuade policy makers from continuing to place heavy restrictions on injecting drug use. In closing this chapter, we examine how unhealthy health-related laws, policies and practices worsened the suffering of illegal drug users.

The starting point in assessing the adverse impacts of the law and policies on drug users is the criminalization of drug use and the use of incarceration as a means of addressing this behavior. The Report of the Global Commission on Drug Policy (2011), for example, identifies several ways that the War on Drugs fuels the HIV pandemic:

- Fear of arrest drives drug users underground and away from HIV testing and prevention services into high-risk environments.
- Restrictions on the provision of sterile syringes without a doctor's prescription result in increases of multiple-person use of syringes, a known route of HIV and other infectious disease transmission.

The staunch opposition of supporters of the War on Drugs to syringe exchange to prevent the spread of HIV in addicts delayed implementation in many parts of the United States for years. A federal ban on funding for these programs was not removed until 2009. Barriers to the funding and operation of syringe-exchange programs, which have been proven to lower incidence rates of HIV infection, constitute a significant risk on injection drug users.

- Prohibitions or restrictions on opioid substitution programs and other evidence-based treatment result in out-of-treatment drug user populations and the spread of HIV disease.
- The heavy costs of the War on Drugs rob monies needed for drug treatment and HIV-prevention programs. As Dwight Eisenhower, who warned of the ever-growing threat of the military-industrial complex, also aptly noted almost 60 year ago, "Every gun that is made, every warship launched, every rocket fired, signifies in the final sense a theft from those who hunger and are not fed, those who are cold and are not clothed" (Eisenhower 1953); to this, he could have added every dollar spent on eradication, interdiction, and arrest related to drug flows is a theft from those in need of drug treatment.

According to the National Institute on Drug Abuse, the institute within the National Institutes of Health that supports scientific research on drug issues and reports its intramural and extramural findings to Congress and the American people:

Addiction is defined as a chronic, relapsing brain disease that is characterized by compulsive drug seeking and use, despite harmful consequences. It is considered a brain disease because drugs change the brain; they change its structure and how it works. These brain changes can be long lasting and can lead to many harmful, often self-destructive, behaviors (National Institute on Drug Abuse 2012).

Whether or not one believes this is an adequate definition, it is certainly noteworthy that drug-research scientists view addiction as a public-health issue involving a compulsive disease that seems most inappropriately "treated" by incarceration. Incarceration, in fact, is harmful to the mental and physical health of drug users, promoting depression, exposure to stress and trauma, and increasing the risk for multiple diseases and disorders (Bingswanger 2010). Ironically, the physical-health and mental-health risks of incarceration, including risk of violence, have been heightened by the increase in conviction for drug-related violations resulting in severe overcrowding in the American penal system.

While drug treatment is available to (some) inmate populations, prisoners commonly endure long waits to begin drug therapy because of staff shortages and limited resources according to research by the Government Accountability Office (2012). Furthermore, assessment of prison-based drug treatment programs reveals significant limitations, including inadequate staffing, wide variation in staff competence and commitment, poor screening practices, comingling of individuals with quite different drug-abuse problems and degrees of drug dependency, lack of prioritization of individuals most in need of drug treatment, inconsistency in program content, significant limits on access to individual one-on-one counseling, wide variation in staff/participant relations, the inclusion of treatment staff with a negative attitudes toward inmates and toward drug treatment, lack of perceived trust among inmates about sharing personal information in group counseling sessions, widespread concern among participants that they can be removed from treatment for small infractions of prison rules, and failure to develop post-release aftercare programming in the community (Correctional Association of New York 2011). The overall adverse impact of incarceration is suggested by findings from a study by Weaver and Lerman (2010) on the relationship between contact with the criminal justice system and social attitudes. They found that even after controlling for other important variables, interaction with the criminal-justice system was a significant predictor of civic and political disengagement and mistrust of government.

Outside of the incarceral setting, access to drug treatment, as a result of government funding and other policies is a fundamental issue in drug-user health. Most drug-treatment programs incorporate 12-step programming, even though they have been found not to be effective for many people. Methadone and buprenorphine maintenance, which have comparatively good track records as drug-treatment methodologies for opioid addiction, are usually isolated from mainstream health care in resource-limited (and often somewhat hidden) opioid replacement clinics (Bourgois 2003a). If addiction were seen and actually treated as a disease like any other, its care would be integrated into health-care systems generally rather than isolated and treated as if the people who suffer from it were contagious or a social risk. Moreover, drug treatment would be comprehensive, low threshold, and be focused on the full reintegration of patients back into the community, features that tend to be lacking in the existing underfunded, under supported treatment "system."

Existing policing practices in many cities involve the confiscation of syringes from drug users. As a result, syringes may not be available at a time of drug craving, and drug injectors may avoid carrying their "works" with them, resulting in the multiple-person use of drug equipment. In our respective interviews with drug injectors, we have found this pattern of policing behavior reported by many drug injectors. Multiple-person use of syringes is known to be a primary source of HIV transmission as well as the spread of other infectious diseases among injection drug users. A similar pattern occurs with crack pipes as well, which, when used by more than one individual, can transmit hepatitis C (Tortu et al. 2004). In a similar vein, condoms, a proven preventive for HIV transmission, may be treated when found on a person by the police as evidence for involvement in commercial sex, leading to a loss of condom availability at times of need among commercial sex workers, who have disproportionate rates of HIV infection. In a report issued by Human Rights Watch (2012) based on detailed interviews with more than 300 commercial sex workers and transgendered people in San Francisco, New York, Los Angeles, and Washington, D.C. (among the urban areas hardest hit by HIV disease) found frequent reports that police officers regularly harassed, threatened, and arrested them for carrying condoms, which police used as evidence of involvement in prostitution. In San Francisco, this practice occurred despite a city law that explicitly banned the use of condoms as evidence of criminal activity. Our own studies in Miami (cf. Needle et al. 2003) found similar police practices on a male sex worker stroll in East Little Havana.

Drug overdose has surpassed HIV infection as a cause of mortality among drug users. There is, however, a safe, nontoxic drug, naloxone, that can quickly reverse opioid overdose and prevent most overdose fatalities. The War on Drugs interferes with saving overdose victims in two ways. First, because witnesses to overdose, usually other drug users, fear prosecution, they often avoid calling for help until it is too late to save the overdose victim. Second, because the War on Drugs reinforces the idea that making naloxone available over-the-counter or with opioid prescriptions would somehow encourage drug use, the antidote is available only through harm-reduction programs like syringe exchanges or in some state programs targeted at drug users. Underlying the War on Drugs approach is a war on harm-reduction strategies that could lower the risk of disease, injury, and death among drug users.

Although it is widely assumed that the popularity of more potent stimulants like crack cocaine and crystal methamphetamine lead to the police crackdowns on these drugs as part of the larger War on Drugs, some research has suggested that the appeal of these drugs may have been a product of the

War on Drugs. When law enforcement targets the drug supply, the most powerful and highly concentrated forms of drugs become more attractive to sellers and users alike, as smaller quantities are easier to hide from police inspection. This pattern also was seen during Prohibition, with stronger forms of alcohol like moonshine displacing weaker drinks like beer. More potent drugs, as we have indicated in Chapter 2, however, increase the risk for overdose and addiction.

CONCLUSION

As we have seen, the health of drug users has not been a primary concern of legal and criminal-justice institutions. On the contrary, these institutions have promoted the darkest images of drug users, portraits that justify their marginalization, arrest, and incarceration. The law, in short, in its many expressions from drug bans, sentencing structures, the War on Drugs, and policing practices has been a primary force in the Othering of drug users in society. Various laws and policies, which appear to critics to be expressions of an attitude of judgment and condemnation, or at least hostile indifference, have burdened the lives of drug users helping to insure high rates of illness, shorter than average life spans, and ongoing social suffering. At the same time, these laws and policies and the availability of drug users as objects of opprobrium and blame provides social justification for multiple social institutions and their employees' social roles, public and private, as well as the considerable expenditure of public funds. The usefulness of the useless is deeply etched in all aspects of the criminal justice and public policy apparatus.

CHAPTER SEVEN

Drug Users in Social Science
The Others We've Made

L
ike prohibitionists, politicians, writers, correctional-institution admin-istrators, movie directors, television producers, and law-enforcement officials, social scientists also have had uses for the Cultural Others who use drugs. This chapter describes how social and behavioral scientists use addicts and drug users under three broad domains: (1) studies of the use of exotic drugs, (2) studies of drug use in social deviance, and (3) studies of people at risk of health problems because of drug use. These arenas of study may overlap, although, for example, the investigation of exotic patterns of drug use tends to be separate from the other two, and the actual number of studies is far less numerous. We address these domains in this order. The first involves discovery of the range of human variation through seeking out extremely distinctive cultural traditions of drug use—very much the province of anthropology, with famous proponents including Richard Evans Schultes, Weston La Barre, and Marlene Dobkin de Rios. Their contributions have given drug researchers perspective on how variable the use of drugs can be in the full breadth of the human condition, including unusual uses of seemingly familiar drugs such as alcohol and tobacco. The drug studies of the second domain, in which the focus is on deviance in social context, have attempted to explain why people use drugs that are socially disapproved or illegal. These studies attend to questions of etiology of drug use and the contextual conditions that appear to nurture it. Notable quantitative proponents of this area of research include Kandel, Brook, Johnston, and O'Malley. Qualitative proponents include Agar, Sterk, and many others. The third domain of drug studies concentrates on the health risks and other risks incurred by drug users, attempting to find ways to prevent the ill effects of drugs. Proponents of this pathway include Booth, McCoy, and numerous others. Each domain will receive attention in this chapter, with some commentary on the political economy and its influence on the direction of research since the inception of the National Institute on Drug Abuse.

The Social Value of Drug Addicts: The Uses of the Useless, by Merrill Singer and J. Bryan Page, 181–204.

DRUG RESEARCH OTHER THAN TREATMENT STUDIES

In studies of people who use drugs in culturally distinctive contexts, social science use of the Cultural Other involves emphasizing the myriad ways that humans seek and interpret altered states. Such studies form distinctive cases that reflect the universal quest among human beings to find meaning and predictability in life through ritual that involves drug use. The second social science use of the Cultural Other serves highly varied agendas, from defining deviance to determining how best to deal with the existence of drug users in society (e.g., issues of policy, criminality, etc.). The last social science use of the Cultural Other focuses on public health and delineates the epidemiology and etiology of diseases that co-occur with drug use (or, in the case of overdose, are directly caused by drug use), and how to respond effectively to them. In short, the social sciences construct three somewhat different but overlapping drug-using Cultural Others: the drug user as cultural actor and knowledge seeker; the drug user as a deviant threat to society; and the drug user as a vulnerable person in need of unforced harm-reduction intervention. Critical to the alternative construction of drug users within particular social sciences has been the intersection of place of use and drugs being consumed, as discussed in the following sections.

EXOTIC DRUG USE

More than the other social sciences, anthropology has dominated the literature on drugs not commonly used in Western society (Singer 2012). Because anthropologists go to out-of-the-way places to study the full range of variability of the human condition, the likelihood of finding people in those places who use lesser-known drugs is high. This likelihood is especially great in ecological zones where there is significant biodiversity. Consequently, anthropologists who study people in jungle habitats often have seen people using drugs that would be deemed exotic from a Western experiential perspective. Schultes (1993), for example, purposely sought people in deep Amazon and its tributaries because he recognized the limitless potential for discovery of new drugs. Anthropological training helps to assure that the observant fieldworker will fully describe encountered drug use and the physical setting and social environment in which it occurs. Moreover, historically, anthropologists were trained to pay special attention to cultural behaviors that differed from Western patterns, making "exotic drug use" an immediate object of interest.

In their focus on the relatively rare and exotic patterns of how humans use drugs, investigators such as Peter Furst, Johannes Wilbert, Richard Evans Schultes, Marlene Dobkin de Rios, and Weston LaBarre adhered to anthropological modes of observation in which they reported cultural context as they saw it from their own respective vantage points and, in light of cultural relativist sentiments within the discipline, generally avoided judging whether what they saw was good or evil. The tone of their publications, however, is not just a product of the culturally nonjudgmental position taken during their time in the field, but in most instances, the people studied by these anthropologists were using drugs that are not associated with addiction or other notable signs of individual or social harm. For example, the peyote use studied by LaBarre (1975 [1938]) took place in the context of a pan-Native American religious movement. In that cultural context, congregants chewed peyote buttons (*Lophophora williamsii*) in order to enter into the visions that allowed them to speak to spirit helpers. In many groups, spirit helpers are essential to receiving spiritual guidance in both mundane and special life circumstances. The mescaline in peyote facilitates these visions as the devotees seek them in the course of ritual, but, in the view of Native American Church members, to have such visions outside of this specific context is highly undesirable. Furthermore, not all congregants are in need of immediate contact with their spirit helpers on the occasion of a specific church service. The peyote experience itself has little to recommend it other than the visions it can produce. The buttons have a violently bitter taste, and the most common immediate reaction to ingesting peyote is to vomit. LaBarre's defense of the Native American Church and its use of peyote in ritual began a decades-long struggle to legitimize use of the drug in this very specific context in response to government efforts to ban peyote as part of broader drug-prohibition efforts. A later statement, published in *Science,* reiterated LaBarre's support of the Native American Church's ritual use of peyote (LaBarre et al. 1951). In this announcement, LaBarre and several other anthropologists who had studied peyote use ethnographically stressed that within the context of the Native American Church peyote

> does not excite, stupefy, or produce muscular in-coordination; there is no hangover; and the habitual user does not develop any increased tolerance or dependence. As for the immorality that is supposed to accompany its use, since no orgies are known among any Indian tribes of North America, the charge has as much validity as the ancient Roman accusation of a similar nature against the early Christians.

Notably, as a result of such efforts, in 1970, the Comprehensive Drug Abuse Prevention and Control Act specifically excluded bans on peyote use by members of the Native American Church:

> The listing of peyote as a controlled substance in schedule I does not apply to the nondrug use of peyote in bona fide religious ceremonies of the Native American Church, and members of the Native American Church, so using peyote are exempt from registration. Any person who manufactures peyote for or distributes peyote to the Native American Church, however, is required to obtain registration annually and comply with all other requirements of the law (Knipe 1995:402).

Nevertheless, a ruling written by Antonin Scalia in 1990 reflecting a 6 to 3 vote by the US Supreme Court stated that two Native American Church members could be denied unemployment benefits because they had been fired for using peyote. Legal protections that apply to ritual use apparently do not extend to the arena of keeping a job (Knipe 1995). LaBarre's advocacy, and the contributions of other anthropologists who have studied peyote use and defended this behavior by members of the Native American Church, while ultimately largely successful, constitutes a rare example of drug users' use of drugs being the beneficiary of social-science writing.

Peter T. Furst (1972, 2006) very thoroughly characterized the patterns of peyote use as practiced among the Huichol of central Mexico. For a period of 35 years, Furst focused largely on Huichol practices related to the ritual use of this drug. While his intent was to describe and analyze this practice, he unintentionally created the opportunity for people presenting themselves as Huichol shamans to charge new-age tourists who read or heard about his work a fee to replicate the Huichol version of the peyote experience. His vivid and convincing accounts of the process of hunting and collecting peyote buttons, performing required ceremonies of administration, and taking the drug have led many adventure- and spiritual-growth hungry North Americans to seek the insights experienced by Furst's Huichol informants. This phenomenon has re-occurred in several instances where shamanistic practices attracted attention because they were associated with use of little-known psychotropic drugs (e.g., ayahuasca use in Peru).

Although Schultes (1938) also weighed in on the issue of peyote, most of his output simply helped to communicate to the rest of the world the variable and elaborate ways of using drugs practiced by people living outside the thrall of Western civilization (cf. Schultes 1976; 1993). By the time of his death in 2001, he had become the foremost ethnobotanical expert on patterns of mind-altering drug use in non-Western societies. His focus in these endeavors was on the plants and their properties, rather than the cultural contexts in which they were used, but he still succeeded in documenting ceremonial rites and customs surrounding the use of plant medicines and psychotropic drugs in various cultural settings. His writings, like Furst's for peyote, may have contributed to the eventual development of touristic quests to experience the effects of ayahuasca, but there is no evidence of direct linkage between Schultes' work and these quests. His own use of exotic drugs during his field research, however, is well documented.

Much more immediate links between drug tourism and specific publications can be found in the case of Marlene Dobkin de Rios's writings about ayahuasca as a tool for healing (Dobkin de Rios 1970; 1971; 1972a; 1972b; 2005). In describing the healing ceremonies conducted by mestizo curanderos, Dobkin de Rios cited the most important city in the region, Iquitos. In present-day Iquitos, tourists who arrive from North America or Western Europe have many options for experiencing the effects of concoctions made of the *Banisteriopsis caapi* vine, either recruiting a "guide" on the street who for a fee will introduce a tourist to a "shaman," or pre-arranging a "shamanism program," consisting of four days of activities in which the tourist may

> Discover shamanism in the Peruvian Amazon. Learn about the amazing healing power of medicinal plants and be part of the magic rituals performed by the Master Shaman. [And, describing a photo on the web site:] The Ayahuasca Rite participants gather at Master Shaman's to prepare the magic circle (Paseos Amazónicos 2013).

Page's former students have made the trip to Iquitos and either enlisted a "shaman" to guide them through an experience of using ayahuasca, or observed other tourists in the process of recruiting a guide for the purpose of finding a "shaman." In Iquitos, Singer has seen brochures for ayahuasca experiences displayed along with other "things to do" information in local hotels and observed lacquered slices of *Banisteriopsis caapi* vine for sale by souvenir vendors.

These activities of experience-seeking by people whose interest in drugs is far from academic seem to be unexpected consequences of serious anthropologists' work. Schultes or Dobkin de Rios would hardly have encouraged people to seek out their informants and take the drugs being studied. The fact that shamanistic tourism has evolved in the vicinity of Iquitos indicates that some drug uses are taken on voluntarily by the users in collaboration with the experience seekers. In these specific cases, the form taken by the "shamanism program," which includes explanations and enactments of the rituals surrounding ayahuasca use, speaks to a desire by the experience-seeking consumer to learn something about the cultural context in which the congregants drink the potion. Authenticity of this cultural experience may not be high, but it leaves the customer satisfied that he/she has attained new insights by means of drug use in an appropriately nurturing environment. The teacher, in turn, makes money, although it is not clear just how lucrative these activities are over time. Economics aside, in transcultural exchanges, ayahuasca instructors encounter what in the past would have been seen as a very unexpected use of drug users.

With regard to the anthropologists' own uses of diverse drug-using populations, it is evident that they profit in several ways from their encounters with drug users:

1. They publish books (which usually bring in modest royalties) and articles that help to establish their reputations as experts on the human behaviors surrounding the use of mind altering drugs..
2. They use their books and articles as justification to obtain further funding for more research, raising their prestige and credibility as researchers on exotic drug use.
3. They are invited to and attend conferences around their respective homelands and beyond to share their findings with academic audiences.
4. They obtain gainful employment on the strength of their research expertise in a relatively rare specialty.
5. Their ongoing productivity in reporting on drug users' activity provides their employers with justification for raising these researchers' salaries.
6. The dissemination of their work to students helps to attract graduate students who wish to pursue related lines of research. This well-educated and highly motivated workforce helps the investigators conduct more research, write more publications, and gain further prestige, funding, and raises in salary.

Clearly, from the informants' point of view, the impact of the data provided to the researchers bestowed on those researchers multiple advantages to which the informants did not necessarily have access. We do not know, in most cases, whether or not the researchers of exotic drug use "gave back" to their informants, although we can surmise that Furst, for example, in his long-term relations with the Huichol,[1] as is the wont of most anthropologists who re-visit people they have studied, effectively engaged in gift-giving and receiving as long-term relationships developed. Perhaps, as also is common, he provided assistance with community initiatives or health problems. The most enmeshed relationship between anthropological drug researcher and informant is Marlene Dobkin de Rios's long-lasting marriage with her key informant, first encountered in the 1960s during her initial field research on ayahuasca (Dobkin de Rios 1970). Unlike key informants of other anthropological researchers, Mr. Rios has had ample opportunity to avail himself of the benefits accrued by his spouse. Nevertheless, regardless of the kind and intensity of reciprocity between researcher and informant, the anthropological researchers on drugs have tended to handle these relations with respect and fairness. Otherwise, they would not have been sustainable for as long as they have endured.

Another anthropologist, Michael Harner, apparently became so enthralled with the role of shamanism in the life of many different small communities that he focused on how shamans approached the spirit world, including in his inquiries the uses of drugs in the practices of shamanism. His early publications (Harner 1973a, 1973b) provided ethnographic reports on how shamans used drugs to gain access to the spirit world, but as his interest in shamanism increased, he published on shamanism as a concept (Harner 1990) and established an institute for the study of shamanism with the idea that people living in modern societies could benefit from shamanistic teachings about the human condition. One of the attractions of this advocacy in favor of shamanism was undoubtedly the appeal of having complete freedom to seek contact with the spirit world by means of drugs. Because in many of the cultural contexts where shamans practice their arts, the shamans are the only people encouraged to use drugs, Harner's particular approach to these people qualifies as a use of drug users.

NOT "EXOTIC," BUT DIFFERENT

Some researchers have focused on drugs that are well known to the Western world, but have very different applications and meanings in non-Western cultural contexts. Johannes Wilbert (1972), for example, characterized the use of tobacco among the Warao of Venezuela in a shamanic tradition of healing and divination. Far from being an everyday drug for general public consumption, tobacco as it was used among the Warao at the time of his field studies was wrapped into large potent cigars and the smoke inhaled. Shamans were the individuals entrusted with the power imparted by tobacco intoxication to have visions. Elaborate ritual supported by origin legends in which tobacco had a role provided context for the use of potent tobacco preparations to elicit mystical visions.

This pattern of use contrasts so radically with the forms of tobacco consumption found in most of the rest of the world, dominated by industrially produced cigarette smoking, that it raises the question: how did tobacco use become a widespread addictive drug if its putative origins were so ritually restricted? First, the process of diffusion from Native Americans to Europeans took the approach of transmitting a trade good that the recipients were free to use however they pleased. The Native Americans who shared the first twists of tobacco with European newcomers did not bother to explain how the Europeans should use it in ritual terms. Techniques of smoking, chewing, and snuffing were demonstrated briefly, and the Europeans soon understood that they had been taught the basics about the ultimate consumer good—one that you not only have to use up as you use it, but one that also makes the consumer want more. The traditional ritual accompaniments to tobacco smoke, whether or not the Native Americans tried to teach them, were largely ignored. The subsequent three centuries saw the rapid diffusion of tobacco throughout the known world (Page 1999:54). The tobacco preparations that spread so rapidly, however, tended to demand caution on the part of the consumer. A pipe or cigar smoker had to avoid inhaling the potent fumes of these apparatuses so as not to become nauseous. A tobacco chewer had to spit out the juice regularly to avoid overdose of nicotine. Snuff, because of the tiny amounts used at a time, provided something of a model for mundane tobacco use, but it was inconvenient in some ways—it induced sneezes and generated the need to manage the production of excess mucus—among others. As we mentioned in Chapter 2, tobacco underwent a process of toning down the amounts of nicotine imparted to the consumer in order to provide a regular, comforting effect without danger of inadvertent overdose. The first hand-rolled, mass produced cigarettes emerged in 1802 in Spain (Goodman 1993), and the future of tobacco consumption was set. Cigarettes took a form that carried little risk of overdose, but delivered a solid dose of addictive nicotine in a convenient, easy-to-use package. Billions have been manufactured since then, and the medical consequences of their consumption have been staggering, with millions of human beings dying of the cancer, emphysema, heart disease, and other ills directly caused by cigarette smoking.

It is difficult to imagine such a complex of consumption and death arising from a ritually circumscribed pattern of tobacco use such as that practiced by the Warao, or for that matter by the Crow (Lowie 1919; 1983) in the context of their highly ritualized cultivation, harvesting, and smoking of tobacco. In the latter case, the use of tobacco smoke among the Crow was also exclusive and confined to ritual contexts, although "ordinary" non-shamans were permitted to smoke on special occasions. What happened with tobacco was the historic and political economic alteration of a drug initially used for controlled ritual objectives into a highly profitable commodity, with users being transformed by Big Tobacco from participants in culturally meaningful ritual practice into addicted and increasingly diseased sources of vast profit. While it does not involve othering (indeed it is driven by themes of drug use normalization), the contribution of cigarette and other tobacco product consumers to the acquisition of great wealth by tobacco corporations is historically the most glaring misuse of drug users.

Alcohol, by far the most ubiquitous of drugs, received the attention of ethnographers in many parts of the world. In both the highlands and the low-lands of Bolivia, however, Heath (1958; 1976; 1991; 2004) and Carter (1977) have focused on consumption of an alcohol preparation of high potency that tests at 178 proof, or 89 percent ethyl alcohol by volume (Heath 1958), more than twice the potency of the gin that aroused so much commentary in 18th Century England. Bolivians call this preparation *alcohol* (in Spanish, the h is silent), and it is the only drink associated with rituals and fiestas. Both among the Aymara, who occupy much of the high country in Bolivia, and among the Camba, a mestizo group that occupies the lowlands near Santa Cruz, people consume this preparation beyond the point of drunkenness in the context of religious and social rituals. Nevertheless, despite the potency of the preparation and the fact that the rituals during which the drinking occurs inevitably lead to drunkenness, neither Carter nor Heath could find any evidence of drunkenness that was not related to ritual.

Both the Camba and the Kolla (terms used respectively for lowland-ers and highlanders) avoided any drunkenness outside of ritual contexts. Furthermore, the two anthropologists found the rituals in which people drank to be infrequent. Heath (1958) did not report the periodicity of fi-estas in which the Camba drank alcohol, but considering the Camba who drank were Catholic (Protestants tended to be teetotal abstinent), and the liturgical calendar would place religious celebrations not less than six weeks apart (e.g., Epiphany to Lent, and Lent to Easter), the likelihood of back-to back, fiesta-driven bouts of drunkenness would be low. Key saints' days and local holidays might change these intervals somewhat, but Heath's original descriptions imply that the fiestas were separated from each other by substantial intervals of time. Wakes could occur at any time, but the Camba did not drink on those occasions, perhaps to avoid interfering with the fiestas' timing (Heath 1958:74). Carter commented that it was fairly common in the highlands to see Aymara- or Quechua-speaking people drunk on the road or in the town plaza, leading casual observers to conclude that there existed a population of Kolla drunkards. Further investigation, however, revealed that from week to week, these drunks were different people. Follow-up studies of people involved in specific drinking-linked rituals showed that most people only drank heavily two or three times a year (Carter 1977:105), depending on what rites of passage and other drinking occasions took place in their respective social environments. In neither the Camba nor the Kolla cultural contexts could the two anthropologists discern any chronic drunkenness, alcoholism, or other health sequelae resulting from the heavy drinking seen during fiestas or other celebrations, although Carter (1977:104) allowed that more rigorous investigation was needed to ascertain the validity of that assessment.

The importance of these investigations in terms of "Othering" addicts lies in their questioning of the concept of addiction as an inevitable consequence of overuse. Lowie (1919; 1983) and Wilbert (1972) observed highly ritualized consumption of tobacco that was not associated with addiction. Heath (1958; 1976; 1991; 2004), and Carter (1977) forwarded a view of human plasticity that rejected the inevitability of chronic drug-related problems, despite heavy consumption of the most potent preparation—178 proof alcohol. To this day the latter view is controversial, but it hinges on an under-investigated aspect of the human condition—ritual circumscription of drug taking behavior. These anthropologists used a point of view—cultural relativism—that led them to question the assumptions made in various forms of public discourse, including biomedical literature, on how humans consume drugs and what consequences result from that consumption.

As Carter's observations indicate (1977:104), it is possible for inattentive observers to mistake highly visible public drunkenness for highly prevalent public drunkenness, when at any given time, a relatively low proportion of the population is drunk, but somebody somewhere is having a wedding or some other ceremony that requires heavy drinking of *alcohol*. The driver of that particular phenomenon in highland Bolivia was not addiction to alcohol among Aymara people, but the meaning given to drunkenness in a cultural context involving a wide variety of rituals that occurred in the lives of individuals infrequently. The majority of these personal rites *required* participants to become drunk because the alcohol was a ritual object, and its full consumption signified that the ritual had been properly observed. Therefore, the host at such a ritual did everything possible to make sure that all of his/her guests were drunk (Carter 1977:102). In that same cultural tradition, the Aymara viewed drunkenness *outside* of the ritual context as a social impropriety.

When we recall the social commentary on the English gin epidemic of the 1700s and early 1800s, we might question those observations of public drunkenness through Carter's same lens, asking the question, "Were these observable drunks always the same people?" The attribution of alcohol addiction to a large segment of the poor population of London failed to take into account whatever social processes drove drinking and drunkenness in those cultural contexts. The view held by the higher classes in England of drinking behaviors among the poor was, like the view taken by non-indigenous Bolivians of their Aymara countrymen, based on superficial observation and insufficient social characterization. Moreover, such observations, and the moral conclusions they feed, commonly are driven by underlying tensions that concentrate at points of social inequality.

CANNABIS AS A CASE IN POINT

In reaction to the Shafer Report, a government commission document that supported ending marihuana prohibition and adopting other methods to discourage use (Shafer et al. 1972), the executive branch of the United States Federal Government initiated studies of Cannabis use in countries where the populations that consumed the drug had done so for decades prior to the initiation of the study. The reasoning (commonly attributed to John Mitchell) that led to this initiative held that if people have been using a drug for a very long time, they are very likely to have experienced negative consequences. In the United States, the widespread use of Cannabis had only six years' time depth in 1972. Therefore, the population of users in the United States did not have enough experience with the drug to have incurred the serious adverse effects that surely (according to Mitchell) accompanied long-term use. Thus, to learn about those effects, investigators had to study populations that had been using Cannabis for at least ten years. The National Institutes of Health issued an announcement in 1972 that was aimed at funding at least three studies of populations that had used Cannabis for a minimum of ten years. Three investigators at the University of Florida, William E. Carter, Wilmer J.

Coggins, and Paul L. Doughty, proposed to conduct a study of the effects of Cannabis among male users in San José, Costa Rica. This project began in the summer of 1973.

In studying the consequences of long-term marihuana use among working-class men in Costa Rica, some of the same inter-class dynamics like those seen in Bolivia and 18th century England became evident (Carter et al. 1980). Newspaper accounts, conversations with health and law enforcement officials, and the political discourse portrayed marihuana users as denizens of the underworld, where questionable morals and illegal activities held sway. When the research team in Costa Rica encountered active marihuana smokers in the working-class barrios, they found a mix of steady skilled workers and small business owners, as well as shady characters and street men who lived by their wits (True et al. 1980). There was a grain of truth in the stereotypic descriptions of marihuana users as they appeared in Costa Rican public discourse of the 1970s, because some marihuana users and dealers encountered by the field team admitted making their living by sneak thievery, small-scale marihuana sales, and a variety of swindles. As the research progressed, however, the networks of informal social relations among the users and dealers led to individuals who were gainfully employed in legitimate endeavors, including building construction, taxi driving, vegetable vending, shoemaking, bread baking, and manufacture of clothing, among other working-class occupations (True et al. 1980). Furthermore, the "stable smokers," as they were labeled in research-team publications, were more numerous than the "street movers." Thus, the planned "Othering" of marihuana users in Costa Rica broke down under ethnographic scrutiny. Again, William E. Carter had conducted an anthropological study of a pattern of drug use that received much social disapproval and found that the rationale for that disapproval had little basis in fact.

The deconstruction of Costa Rican prejudice against working-class marihuana users was not simply a product of the research team's working so closely with study participants that the process affected how the study team perceived marihuana users and marihuana use. The entire Costa Rica study of marihuana use was designed to uncover negative effects on health and well-being of very long-term marihuana users. Consequently, most of the study's research procedures were selected and designed to test hypotheses in the areas in which long-term Cannabis use was suspected to cause problems with, specifically lung function, vision, sleep electroencephalography, serum testosterone, psychomotor function, and cognitive function. Local physicians and technicians conducted all tests, and were blinded to whether or not the study participants used or did not use marihuana. Results of users were unproductively compared with results of matched controls.[2]

Despite the findings of the Costa Rica (Carter et al. 1980) and Jamaica (Rubin and Comitas 1975) studies, both of which, like the Shafer report (Shafer et al. 1972), failed to find causal relations between marihuana smoking and criminality or health problems, the popular press and political discourse continued to assert that marihuana use should be banned in the United States and marihuana users should be punished and vilified (Nahas 1973).[3] The reason for this persistence of negative perception of marihuana is based not at all on new scientific findings about the acute and long-term effects of marihuana use. Rather, the negative perception was attributable primarily to the fact that in 1975, the North American voters who opposed changing marihuana laws still outnumbered (albeit narrowly) advocates of changing these prohibitory laws. Combined with a factor that Page (1997) has called "strongly held beliefs," that is especially rampant among politicians who do not bother with scientific findings, the voters' negative opinions about marihuana still carried the day in 1975. Moreover, treating marihuana use harshly emerged as a political strategy that politicians could use to show voters they were "tough on crime" or were helping to protect society from a slide into moral iniquity, a strong fear among a vocal segment of the American population.

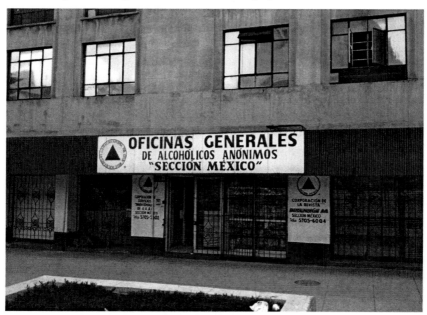

Alcohol treatment in Mexico (Photo by Elyse Singer)

In the case of anthropologists' studies of Cannabis smokers, the investigators set out to make one use of them (i.e., negative models to support US drug policies) but found that use—to provide evidence that marihuana smoking is bad for marihuana smokers—failed to yield the "desired" evidence.[4] Instead, the participants in the Costa Rica study gave evidence on just how difficult it was to find adverse effects of long-term use, even with the best detection equipment and expertise.

POLICY AGAINST SCIENCE

The Costa Rica case exemplifies a tension that has exerted influence on the pursuit of scientific understanding in the field of drug use and its consequences. The government's desire to declare that drugs (meaning everything except the "legal" ones) are harmful has led to intensified pursuit of scientific evidence that consuming drugs, especially illegal ones like cocaine and heroin, is bad for the consumers. In its highest forms, however, science is not designed to fulfill what is essentially a political agenda. In principle, science seeks explanations of phenomena based on close, unbiased examination of those phenomena. During the latter half of the 20th and early 21st centuries, the tension between policy, apparently formulated on the basis of accumulated attitudes, class and racial prejudices, political stratagems, and some clinical anecdotes, and science continued. Not surprisingly, policy based on bad or misinterpreted information has held sway most of the last 60 years.

Ironically, the politicians who posture as "tough on crime" and "anti-drug" warriors have had a major influence on the availability of funding for scientists seeking to understand drug use. This process has been discernible as a trend since the inception of the National Institute on Drug Abuse (NIDA), the United States' principal agency that funds studies of drug use. The funding available in support of NIDA had a sharp upward trajectory since its inception in 1974, beginning with a few million dollars, reaching $800 million by 2001, and peaking at $1.06 billion in fiscal year 2011 (NIDA Appropriations Table 2013). This figure has hovered around the $1 billion mark since 2003. In the 1980s and 1990s, when most of the major increases in NIDA's budget occurred, either the sitting president was Republican or key Republican members of the House and Senate were in position to exert influence on those appropriations. Apparently, they saw it as in their interest to give generous appropriations to NIDA in pursuit of knowledge about drug use, because that activity gave them credibility as anti-drug warriors.

The irony of this circumstance derives from the fact that the scientists who successfully competed for the funds made available by drug warriors produced findings that did not necessarily reinforce the drug warriors' ideology of drug abuse. Furthermore, the people who helped NIDA decide who received research funding were predominantly scientists whose political sympathies often went to the side of liberal Democrats. Consequently, the formulators of drug prevention programs and community organization programs who had attracted the attention of Nancy Reagan, for example, such as Daytop Village in New York, had difficulty getting favorable scores from initial review groups at NIDA who found these applicants' science weak. Nevertheless, NIDA kept on receiving increased budgets between 1980 and 2001. One consistently funded researcher, James Inciardi, despite being a lifelong Democrat, sheepishly confessed that he had voted for G.H.W. Bush in 1988 in order to assure adequate funding for research on drug use (personal communication to Bryan Page (1989). His thinking, shared to varying degrees by other funded investigators in sociology, anthropology, psychology, and economics, perceived the Republicans as a little more mystified and frightened by illegal drug users than were the Democrats. The Republicans' fear and bewilderment with regard to these threatening Others seemed to produce fatter research budgets than the Democrats' humanitarian view of addicts and addiction. The advent of AIDS and funding to address the epidemic among intravenous drug users (IDUs) changed the funding dynamic somewhat, although the tone of that time was not so much concern for IDUs' health but rather fear of them serving as an HIV "bridge" to "normal" people.

As apparently generous as Republicans were to drug research, however, they were even more so to interdiction and enforcement. Their investment in those efforts, including border patrol, Coast Guard, customs, and AWACS, plus an extravagant "Plan Colombia" costing billions throughout the 1980s and '90s. The DEA alone received a little over twice as much money as NIDA during the budget years of 2008–2012 (Drug Enforcement Agency 2013). "Plan Colombia," a collaboration between the US and Colombian governments to stop traffic in cocaine and heroin, cost over $500 million per year all by itself between 2001 and 2005. Without question, the appropriations for interdiction have been far greater than for research on drug abuse and one product of that distribution of funds is the demonization of drug users as menacing threats that merit the considerable expenditure of tax dollars.

This point aside, it is clear that monies for research on drug use and drug users were available on a fairly steep growth curve before 2004. When compared to other institutes in the National Institutes of Health, NIDA between

2000 and 2012 had larger allocations than 14 of the 26 other institutes, some of which dealt with much more widespread and serious problems than drug abuse. For example, the National Institute of Alcohol Abuse and Alcoholism received about half as much money per year as NIDA during that period (National Institutes of Health 2013). Given the massive negative impact of alcohol on the population of the United States, this disproportion seems counterintuitive. The NIDCR, an agency for dental and craneo-facial health received only about $400 million in 2012, about 40 percent of what NIDA received in the same year. The National Institute on Aging (NIA) receives roughly the same allocation that NIDA receives to attend to the scientific investigation of aging, the most pervasive health issue of all.

To say that social and behavioral scientists, including both authors of this book, have benefitted disproportionately from NIDA's rapid growth in allocations would be an understatement. One of the most striking features of socio/behavioral research is its cost, and because the principal nexus of drug use as a health problem is human behavior, the scientific questions about drug use that arise from the social/behavioral area are myriad. Much of the research conducted under NIDA's auspices has been, therefore, expensive. Whether one is trying to understand patterns of drug-using behavior or attempting to prevent uptake of drug use or seeking to improve addiction treatment, research on drug use is costly. People being tested, interviewed, or intervened with often require extensive contact with professional interviewers, medical staff, field recruiters, and participant observers, all of whom require salary or wages to perform their research functions. These salaries constitute the bulk of very large budgets that successful grant applications contain. A grant funded by NIDA to conduct social and/or behavioral research can easily cost $200,000 or more per year in direct costs, with indirect costs adding 50 percent to the grant's total budget. Grants costing $500,000 per year (direct cost) in this context are not uncommon, and often 90 percent or more of those costs go to paying the collectors and analysts of data. Research grants in which most of the investigation takes place in a laboratory, because staffing needs are not heavy, tend not to cost nearly as much as social/behavioral field-based studies.

A successful applicant for NIH funds to conduct a study of drug-using behavior can find him- or herself managing large sums of grant funding, which enhances the investigator's status in his/her home institution, and, as the study's results are published, the scientific community at large. The availability of drug users in various states—active users in street environment, active users who are seeking treatment for addiction, recovering users in treatment, or post-treatment recovering users—determines whether or not the investigator can propose and conduct the projects that bring money, employees, prestige, and academic fame. Social/behavioral scientists, then, have considerable incentive to put drug users of all sorts to use as study participants. How the investigators write about these participants is highly variable in terms of descriptors, analytic conclusions, emergent information, and living context. Writers such as Denise Kandel and Judith Brook, who specialized in cross-sectional and longitudinal surveys that included both drug users and non-users, wrote in broad terms of risk and vulnerability over time:

> The findings that drug use continued to be a predictor of psychiatric disorders—independent of overlapping variance with the subjects' initial psychiatric disorders—adds [sic] considerable important information. First, it helps to rule out the possibility that the drug use was epiphenomenal, in the sense of being a reaction to, or otherwise determined by the individual's psychiatric disorder. It is likely that the adverse effects of drug use on psychiatric disorders tend to accumulate during the individual's development (Brook et al. 1998:328–329).

> Our study examined predictors of smoking initiation among nonsmokers and progression to daily smoking among smokers over a 1-year interval by race/ethnicity in a national longitudinal sample of adolescents (mean age = 15 years). A distinguishing feature of our investigation was the simultaneous consideration of individual characteristics, proximal social influences, and broader contextual factors that index both school characteristics and state policies toward cigarette smoking as predictors of smoking behaviors within a statistical approach that took the hierarchical nature of the data into account. This approach identifies potential interdependence among adolescents within schools and within states that would be ignored in more traditional single-level approaches (Kandel et al. 2004:133).

In both of these brief excerpts, the investigators are using discrete variables collected from both drug users and non-users that they hypothesize to be related to each other. Their goal is to predict co-occurrence of variables of interest. These uses of drug users contrast in terms of method and style with the writings of those whose research focused on developing an understanding of why people use drugs, using a participant observation methodology:

Since he excelled at everything within his reach and had too much energy to keep off the streets, it was only a question of time before Tito [pseudonym] began abusing the drugs that flood U.S. inner cities. Youths embracing street culture often bond with one another around drugs. It is almost impossible to escape them (Bourgois 1997:28).

The study participants testified that intense social pressure played no more than a moderate part in their decisions to use illegal drugs. Most (two-thirds of all illegal drug users) said that their principal reason for beginning a specific drug was that their friends made it look attractive to them. This evidence does not confirm the notion that unscrupulous street denizens lure good children into the world of drug use. Those who use are already motivated to do so, and those who give them opportunities to use for the first time do not necessarily have anything to gain by these invitations (Page 1990:182).

If nothing else this book [a life history of a street drug user] seeks to present Tony [one active user] as I have come to know him—a man like myself with heartfelt hopes and fears, struggling to make it in a world that is often harsh, regularly indifferent, and at times life threatening. If Tony as a living, breathing, thinking, and hurting person were kept in mind in every policy discussion about what to do about the "drug problem," I suspect that we would come up with far better "solutions" than those that guide contemporary actions from the failed War on Drugs to the far less than adequate (and far less than systematic) drug treatment "system" (Singer 2006:11).

All three of these narratives reflected perspectives on the phenomenon of drug use and drug users based on a combination of participant observation and in-depth interviewing. Rather than citing an array of discrete contextual factors, they relied for their perspective on drug use on a contextual gestalt derived from hours spent with drug users by researchers on street corners, alleyways, and abandoned buildings in inner city locations.

However these investigators approached the phenomena associated with drug use, they all depended at their core on access to people who used drugs. In that sense, every kind of social/behavioral scientist who studies drug-use etiology, epidemiology, treatment, or prevention has a use for drug users. These individuals, equipped with advanced degrees in their disciplinary specialties, have built careers based on their access (and ability to gain access) to populations of drug users, win grants to recruit them into studies and get raises and promotions on the basis of the reports published about the users' entry into drug use, treatment for addiction, support of drug-using networks, and inculcation of new drug users, among other topics. This statement is not intended to pass judgment on the people who study drug users as exploitative users of drug users (carrying out such research is our own profession too after all), but rather it emerges from an examination of uses in various endeavors. We, as authors, came through the process of characterizing other forms of use, to the realization that we are included in the group of people who have use for drug users as participants in our studies and by extension, providers of wherewithal to further our careers.

In most instances of social/behavioral scientists' use of drug users, the efforts of the researchers were dedicated to discovering principles that could help addicts in their struggles with addiction, or prevent young people from becoming addicted, or reduce the risk of health consequences of drug use. Some studies have resulted in direct benefits to the participants, as in Singer's work on mitigating risk and harm among IDUs in Hartford's Puerto Rican Community (Singer 1993; 1996a) or addressing other health risks of drug users (Grau et al. 2009, Singer 1996b) or Page and colleagues' (2006) classification of injection implements by measurement of contamination. In the latter study, the field team shared the findings from the laboratory that cookers (receptacles for mixing drugs with water) had very high levels of HIV contamination (counts in excess of 100,000 copies per mm^3) as soon as the results were available.

The examples cited above, however, are relatively small in scale and involve relatively few drug users compared to the large-scale studies in schools conducted by Gilbert Botvin (Epstein and Botvin 2002; Lynne-Landsman et al. 2011) and his colleagues or Howard Kaplan (Liu and Kaplan 2001). Studies of this nature are very costly because of their scale, and their results are featured in reports of the responsible funding agencies. They in fact receive much more attention than the smaller studies that use ethnographic methods to characterize drug use. The quintessential large-scale study in NIDA's portfolio is the perennial series of surveys conducted by Lloyd Johnston and colleagues called Monitoring the Future (e.g. Johnston et al. 1985, 1986). The results of this survey often become fodder for political statements about success or failure of national drug policy.

THE BUREAUCRATIC LANDSCAPE

How social and behavioral science uses drug users has a landscape that was shaped in the early 1970s as the National Institutes of Health configured agencies specializing in alcohol problems, drug abuse, and mental health. Most of the bureaucrats in those agencies at the level of project officer or higher have advanced background in social/behavioral science, and they also have uses for drug users. The studies that populate their portfolios for extramural funding focus on drug users who must be identified, characterized, and/or treated as part of their investigations. The present array of agencies, including NIAAA, NIDA, and NIMH, can trace its configuration to a paper published by Robert Dupont (1974) the first director of NIDA. He was faced with an already entrenched institute (NIAAA) that focused on alcohol and another (NIMH) that focused on mental health. Furthermore, the recognized most dangerous drug, tobacco, was a major focus of the National Cancer Institute. In order to be able to discuss alcohol, tobacco, and drugs in the same discourse, Dupont chose to refer to all of them at once as "substances":

> Alcoholism and drug abuse budgets did not make a significant impact until the 1970s. Because of large increases over the last three years, substance abuse programs taken together now exceed the Federal investment made in all other mental health programs. Initially the Federally funded substance abuse programs were components of the community mental health centers, but recent experience has convinced most experts in these fields that substance abuse programs are sufficiently unique to require separate administrative structures (DuPont 1974:1).

In so doing, Dupont asserted the need for specialization in NIH's approach to "substances." Thereafter, all scientific investigation of "substance" related questions occurred within the framework that Dupont outlined. After 2000, NIDA began providing some funding for tobacco research, primarily in the social/behavioral area, but this has been one of only a few variations from that scientific structure.

Importantly, this domination of drug-research activity is made possible by the effectiveness of NIDA officials in presenting their case to the arms of government that control funding. That case has involved a massive "Othering" of drug users to the Congress and to the general public through self-published monographs with titles such as *Use of Licit and Illicit Drugs by America's High School Students 1975–1984* (Johnston, O'Malley, and Bachman 1985), *Drug Abuse among Minority Youth: Methodological Issues and Recent Research Advances* (De la Rosa and Adrados, eds. 1993), *PCP Phencyclidine Abuse: An*

Appraisal (Petersen and Stillman, eds. 1978), and *Young Men and Drugs in Manhattan: A Causal Analysis* (Clayton and Voss 1981). These and many similar publications suggest that NIDA has sought, ever since its inception, to use the existence of drug users and addicts in furtherance of its agenda to dominate drug research, and establish a kind of hegemony over drug users.[5]

NIDA has demonstrated particular interest in research on networks of informal relations among drug users (cf. Needle et al. 1995). In its 151st research monograph, the agency presented studies that reflect the utility of tracing networks of informal social relations among drug users. NIDA's support of this kind of research, with an orientation toward gaining access to and intervening in the populations of interest to change their behavior, sounds like a parallel with the British Colonial Administration's support of Evans-Pritchard's studies of the Nuer and Dinka in southern Sudan—study of warlike and unruly tribes under British colonial rule to understand better how to "pacify" them. The literature on users of illegal drugs (e.g., Agar 1973; True et al. 1980) suggested that networks among the individuals who rely on friends and acquaintances to identify sources and supplies of drugs could serve as a conduit for identifying active drug users in order to recruit them into studies or otherwise learn about their drug-using behavior. Ongoing access to these networks was also seen by NIDA officials as a potentially valuable way of keeping up with emerging trends in the use of illegal drugs. Subsequent to Monograph #151, further research funded by NIDA (e.g., Koester et al. 2005; Needle et al. 1998) investigated the connections between networks and infection by HIV and Hepatitis C. Although the concept of studying networks started out resembling the British Colonial Authority's targeting of the Nuer in its desire to bring a difficult-to-govern group under heel, most of its applications since 1995 have focused on preventing the spread of blood-borne pathogens. Evans-Pritchard was commissioned by the Colonial Authority to learn as much as he could about the structure of Nuer society and the motivations within that structure for going to war. His inquiries led to an insight about conflict in the context of segmented patrilineages that proved somewhat useful to the Colonial Authority (Evans-Pritchard 1940). Where Evans-Pritchard's studies clearly accrued power to the State (in this case, the British Empire) through improved governing of the Nuer, studies by Trotter, Needle, Koester, and others, led to improvement of health, even though that improvement involved people considered marginal to the State.

None of the preceding assertions would presume to accuse NIDA of having bad intentions toward drug users and addicts. NIDA's interest in drug users' personal networks, for example, stems from a strong desire to prevent the torment of drug abuse in vulnerable populations, or at least prevent some of the most severe consequences. With regard to HIV/AIDS, knowledge of interpersonal networks can identify key individuals whose position in the network makes them ideal participants in intensive interventions to prevent the spread of HIV among peers who self-inject drugs. Efforts to study networks among drug users can identify the pathways for preventing drug use and/or referring users to treatment. Nevertheless, there is more than a taint of hegemonic thinking in the desire to use network studies to find a remedy for the problem of drug use in the United States. Understanding of drug users and their heterogeneity, as delineated by scores of ethnographic studies, guides us toward a rejection of categories of social distinction such as "drug users," or "addicts," or "alcoholics," as an implicitly hegemonic set of terms. Drug users, by definition, use drugs. But some of them also are movie stars, sports celebrities, business executives, social scientists, or stay-at-home parents. Drug use only trumps other social categorizations for some people and not others. Moreover, as noted above, drug use research does not necessarily support our dominant cultural models of drug users or of long-term drug effects. In making this case, social scientists, in fact, actively seek to counter some of the abusive uses of drug users that they witness in society.

Ironically, the steady gains in understanding how people become drug users and the process of addiction as a health phenomenon have tended to blur the lines of demarcation among institutes in NIH. Illegal drug users often commit their most serious crimes under the influence of alcohol (Goldstein et al. 1990). Cocaine users often resort to alcohol to mitigate the "crash" associated with cocaine withdrawal (Page and Míguez-Burbano 1999). Drug users and alcoholics commonly smoke tobacco in conjunction with their use of the other drugs (Singer et al. 2006). What the bureaucratic structure of NIH went to great pains to separate does not remain separate in the real-life encounters between social/behavioral scientists and humans engaged in the behaviors of interest. In the process of training young scientists to conduct funded studies of drug-using behavior, we have repeatedly seen difficulties in conceptualizing proposals and deciding on their most appropriate destinations, because the already-recognized relations among alcohol, tobacco, and other drugs are very enmeshed in the field, but the funding agencies prefer to keep other drugs separate from alcohol. In terms of the study of populations, investigators are asked to keep alcoholics separate from other addicts. It is possible to step across these bureaucratic boundaries, and the phenomenon of the AIDS pandemic represents a good example of this process, with agencies including NIMH, NIDA, NIAAA, and NIAID cooperating and sharing resources in furtherance of understanding and restricting the spread of HIV infection (see Page and Singer 2010: 70-85).

CONCLUSION

The processes that formed the relationship between social and behavioral science and the populations that consume drugs inevitably led to some forms of hegemonic thinking, regardless of the noble intentions of the social and behavioral scientists. This kind of thinking appears to be less prevalent among those researchers who conduct street-level ethnography than among those who organize longitudinal surveys. Both varieties of research are important in understanding content and prevalence of the behaviors that trouble and fascinate us. The first generation of research that combined ethnographic and survey approaches to studying drug users had considerable difficulty in achieving mutually acceptable findings (Page and Singer 2010), but investigators have, under the general rubric of "mixed methods" (e.g., Heckel and Moore 2009; Boeri et al. 2008; Singer et al. 2005) achieved increasingly seamless marriages of the two approaches. This trend appears to us to be the wave of the future in social-science research about drug use. Readers of research results will no longer be satisfied with purely qualitative studies that cannot comment on prevalence of the characterized behaviors, or cannot adequately characterize the behaviors that they quantify. This kind of research will have built into it the perspective that individual human beings, with their contradictions, idiosyncrasies, strengths and frailties inhabit the categories "drug user," or "addict." We hope that this kind of perspective moves all of us—writers, reporters, politicians, bureaucrats, movie-makers, and social/behavioral scientists—to use caution when we speak of these categories.

NOTES

1 See Furst (2006:1) for an explanation of his using this gloss rather than the people's own *Wixáritari* term to denote themselves.

2 See Carter (1980) for a full description of the study design. Given the primitive state of computers in 1973, the study team opted for a matched pair-design to determine the effects of long-term marihuana smoking. A design involving comparison of populations of users and nonusers would be appropriate nowadays, using statistical controls, rather than matching users and nonusers for key variables.

3 We include Nahas (1973) under popular press because his books about marihuana sold fairly well in the early 1970s. He had a pretense of science, as he was an anesthesiologist. Nahas did not, however, gain acceptance in the endeavor of determining the actual effects

of marihuana. He failed repeatedly to win funding from NIH review panels, based on his faulty, agenda-laden science.

4 Of course, none of the scientists "desired" a specific result from their studies, but the original funding impetus had identified the government's agenda in these studies—to find as many as possible negative effects of smoking marihuana. The story circulating in Washington at the time of this initiative was that John Mitchell, in answer to Richard Nixon's distress over the recommendations of the Shafer Report (Shafer et al. 1972), suggested that conducting studies in countries where people had been using Cannabis for a long time would yield convincing negative effects, which in turn would justify keeping marihuana criminalized.

5 This agenda received attention in a paper presented by Page at the AAA meetings in 1993: "To Own the Streets: Implications of Approaches to Studying Drug Use in Dade County, Florida." Paper presented at the annual meetings of the American Anthropological Association, November 17–21, 1993, Washington, DC.

CONCLUSION

From the Making and Using of the Useless to Social Integration

I n his introduction to Polish journalist Ryszard Kapuścibski's book *The Other*, Neal Ascherson (2008:8), observes that "The perception of Otherness, leading to the treatment of the Other as less than human, has been an intra-European habit for millennia, even though it has only just been given a title." Taking this idea a step further, it is probable that the perception of Otherness is a requirement of maltreatment of fellow human beings; the greater the injury inflicted the more demonic the image of the Other. The making of Otherness as social process, as this suggests, is packed with coveting, guilt, and excuse. Our capacity to see fellow human beings as an Other, quite different from "us" or "our" people (with a built-in privileged sense of being the good people, the right and proper people, the intelligent and well-mannered people, the civil and civilized people, the only real people), holds within it the seeds of the grosses forms of inhumanity, as well as diverse varieties of everyday insult, indignity, and insensitivity. Othering, which constitutes a form of social exclusion, is often characterized, by symbolic violence and the naturalization of disadvantage, exploitation and structural, if not outright physical, violence. While it may begin with callousness, Othering can end in holocaust, ethnic cleansing, and genocide.

Kapuścibski, who, influenced by the ideas of Polish anthropologist Bronislaw Malinowski (1922), including the notion that "to judge something, you have to be there," spent his career among Others outside of his native land, outside of Europe, and in, from the Euro-centric perspective, the denigrated regions of the world among people of color. In his travels, Kapuścibski (2008:14) found that each of the individuals he met around the world, "like the rest of us, ... has his joys and sorrows, his good and bad days; he is glad of his successes, does not like to be hungry and does not like it when he is cold; he feels pain as suffering and misery, and good fortune as satisfying and fulfilling." Additionally he stressed, "We treat the Other above all as a stranger (yet the Other doesn't have to mean a stranger), as the representative of a separate species, but the most crucial point is that we treat him as a threat"

The Social Value of Drug Addicts: The Uses of the Useless, by Merrill Singer and J. Bryan Page, 205–218.

(Kapuściþski 2008:58). In other words, Kapuściþski experienced the common humanity, the recognized sense of shared experience, and mutual fear and desire in such encounters, a capacity that runs counter to the tendency to construct Others, and especially to engage in Othering with adverse and painful consequences. As Sabelli (2013:19) points out,

> Kapuściński clearly presents the concept of separation as an unjust, outdated approach to encountering otherness. He believes that we must look for ways of cooperation due to the evolving, multicultural character of today's world.

While Kapuściński has been criticized for essentialism, especially with reference to his book *The Shadow of the Sun,* his writings reflect a commitment to obtaining firsthand experience rather than relying on prevailing stereotypes. Unfortunately, Ascherson emphasizes, in his empathic approach, Kapuściński swam upstream; glumly the flow of human judgments and actions often have been in the opposite direction, as drug users well know from personal everyday experience as outsiders.

Kapuściński's effort to avoid negative Othering was rooted in his affection for the work of philosopher Emmanuel Levinas. Levinas's life overlapped with one of the most grotesque Otherings of history, the Holocaust. Observes Kapuściński (2008:34), "It is ... indifference towards the Other, which creates an atmosphere capable in particular circumstance of leading to Auschwitz...." Otherness, in short, is of consequence, it is the first step on the road that can lead to the kind of massive destruction of human life that characterized the crooked pathway of the 20th century, a period overpopulated with efforts to segment humanity, mislabel some as less than or other than fully human, or not completely sane, or not having any worth or reason for being and hence authorizing their elimination in some fashion. In the case of drug abusers, it has been used to justify and fund an elaborate system of social control that has made the United States the incarceration capital of the world, with four times the historic average penal population of the period before the 1970s and seven times greater than in Western Europe. More precisely, it has been used to rationalize why one-third of African American males under the age of 40 who did not complete high-school are currently locked away behind bars. In America, drug-abuse Othering and mass incarceration have gone hand-in-hand.

As we have tried to show in this book, Othering does not just happen automatically or naturally, it must be manufactured and reinforced across the institutions and communication vehicles within society. To have impact, it must be reproduced and become embedded in the weft and warp of the fabric of society. In this way, it is naturalized and its social construction disguised. A common strategy in this process is the blaming of disparity on the depre- cated. In the case of drug users, victim-blaming is routine and enshrined in public policy. Rather than drug abuse being seen and responded to socially as a faulty coping response to discrimination, abuse, or other forms of struc- tural or symbolic violence, as has been suggested by a considerable body of research, it is popularly portrayed (despite its notable social patterning) as an act of individual choice, personal deviance, lack of moral direction, or other deficit of character and punished accordingly.

Additionally, we have suggested, Othering is purposeful; it has practical benefits. Specifically, it serves interests and rewards its perpetrators. Other- ing, in short, has its advocates, its operators, its benefactors. On whatever avenues of distinction Otherness flows, be they real or invented, grand or miniscule, or even nonexistent (prior to the Othering), or have as their foun- dation cultural, language, behavioral, ethic, regional, social, or other asserted or actual difference, Otherness is not caused by dissimilarity. Humans can live with and even celebrate differences and distinctions. Hence, Othering as a social process need not invent dissimilarity; rather it must assign dis- similitude a meaningful social value. This is achieved by ordering groups of people hierarchically and "continuously producing and re-creating symboli- cally marked 'cultural' [or other] distinctions among them" (Wolf 1982:380).

Reproduction across time and place, as Saïd (1978) stressed, entails identifying and magnifying the alleged weaknesses of the Other, or even a largely imaginary construction of such deficits. In no small measure, Othering also requires forgetting, not seeing, projection, and invention. Conversely, it involves an opposite set of elevations of self that are no less imaginary, embel- lished, blinded, and colored by advantageous misremembering. As noted in the Introduction, these tasks are achieved through the manipulation of words (i.e., drugspeak and the language of oppression) (Gordon 1994, Bosmajian 1983) and images (i.e., circulating visual texts) (Adrian 2003). And they are enforced through policies and actions (e.g., incarceration, shake-downs, street sweeps) that tie image to oppression.

Othering often entails a self-fulfilling prophecy. That which is claimed is created. Rejection by others, for example, is known to cause chronic stress leading in some individuals to the adoption of coping strategies that involve withdrawal and isolation (Link et al. 1997). In this sense, the act of Othering, and what it portends for the object of ridicule and abuse affirms the "soundness" of discriminatory assessment. In the words of Cornel West (1993), Othering inflicts "ontological wounds" on the ostracized, leading to low self-esteem and self-derogation as it is internalized and accepted as valid. As ethnographic researchers, we often encounter very harsh assessments of drug users among drug-using populations. Internalization, the end state of symbolic violence, is fostered by the images and messages of express by the mass media, the courts, the entertainment sector, and other institutions in society.

As we have seen, the Othering process is never uniform nor without sites of contradiction; rather, Othering structures tend to be burdened, in ways small and large, by pieces that do not fit the larger destructive pattern. The existence of contradiction or even resistance, unfortunately, does not necessarily lead to halting the damaging process of Othering. For example, even though racists may have fond feelings for individual denigrated Others in their lives, this does not block them from holding racist sentiments about particular groups or engaging in acts of racial oppression; similarly, the McCarthy-era witch hunt had its vehement critics, and McCarthy himself was not without remarkable contradiction, but people were publically Othered and suffered nonetheless. In the case of drug abusers, it is evident that there are literary, cinematic, social scientific, and other sources that present alternative understandings that call into question the assertions that undergird stigmatization and demonization. This book, of course, has that very intention. The alternative view of drug users stresses several key points:

1. Cultural messages about drug users in the media reflect a simplified worldview of binary opposites composed of the healthy mainstream and its malignant deviants.

2. Public pronouncements about drug users are routinely sensationalized and rely, as Harry Anslinger did in his testimony before the US Congress in support of the Marihuana Tax Act and in his "Marijuana, Assassin of Youth" article, on the cherry picking of extreme cases to typify general patterns of drug-user behavior (Anslinger et al. 1937).

3. Empirical studies of drug users, like those carried out by Carl Hart (2013) and numerous other medical and social science researchers, produce findings that challenge conventional stereotypes about drug users but evidence-based understandings rarely inform public policy on drug use.

4. The public is systematically and purposefully misinformed by the media, other mainstream institutions, and the public statements of politicians and media pundits about drug users and their behavior.

5. Moral panics about new drug scourges sweeping the land or particular vulnerable populations, are revealed, as time passes, to occur independent of actual increases in drug use or strong evidence of significant increases in drug-related threats to health and social welfare.

6. Social crusades targeting particular groups of drug users commonly reflect points of social apprehension and serve to enhance the social control and exploitation of subordinated ethnic, class, gender, or other groups characterized as a threat to the status quo (which although presented as normal and natural is more appropriately typified as the prevailing structure of privilege and social inequality).

The assessment offered in previous chapters is intended to identify some of the ways and cultural places drug users become Others. But the goal is not simply to understand the calculated making of the useless but to imagine and bring into being an alternative to the contemporary pariah status and social misuse of drug users. Our argument is that the starting points for addressing the adverse sides of drug use lies in embracing the Levinasian de-demonization of drug users and their re-incorporation into a more just mainstream society through the investment of resources and the mobilization of human compassion, harm reduction, treatment, and linkage with the resources for sustainable lives. The benefits to society of this dramatic transition, we believe, include an end to the ineffective (at least in terms of official goals) but enormously costly War on Drugs, re-acquisition of forfeited rights and freedoms, enhanced social equality, and diminished (real and imagined) threat from drug consumers. It is not the degree to which we marginalize and condemn drug users that we address "our drug problem" but, on the contrary, the degree to which we avoid such behaviors that we create the social space for achieving this goal. Several studies come to mind that support this assertion.

With funding from the National Institute on Drug Abuse, Singer and colleagues (Dushay et al. 2001) implemented a comparison of two HIV risk reduction intervention models for drug users. One model (which existed in two ethnically specific versions and was implemented by ethnically matched NGOs) was designed, in conjunction with community members, to be culturally targeted to African American and Puerto Rican drug users. The other model was ethnically neutral and was implemented through a drug-treatment program. Findings of the study showed that contrary to our expectations the ethnically targeted models were not particularly more effective with their respective ethnic populations than was the ethnically neutral model with these same populations. Why? Review of these programs in operation suggested that the ethnically neutral model placed a significant degree of emphasis on sensitivity, remaining non-judgmental, and communicating authentic caring for their project clients. This kind of treatment, the inversion of Othering (which can certainly be found at some drug-treatment programs), had a powerful effect: it convinced long-term drug users to change their behaviors to a degree that matched paying keen attention to their ethnic identity in reducing HIV infection risk. In the second study, Singer and co-workers (2001) collected the narratives drug users told each other in the course of daily life acquiring and using drugs. Known on the street as "war stories," these tales cover various topics, such as "learning the ropes" of drug use or making "unexpected valuable discoveries" (e.g., of lost cash or drugs). Among the themes found in this repertoire is one that might be labeled "acts of surprising kindness," in which the storyteller relays an occasion in which someone treated them personally with far greater compassion than they had learned to ever expect on the streets. These events touched their hearts and became part of their cherished and, when the opportunity arose, shared memories. Suggested by these two studies—indeed unanticipated findings of them—is the degree to which people—all people—cherish kindness and respond positively to it. Othering, not surprisingly, has the opposite effects and can, if the opportunity arises, as seen in war zones, produce escalating exchanges of Othering and atrocity.

Although often labeled and treated as useless, if not as incarnations of evil or as threatening burdens on society, drug users, in fact, serve many uses: for others. These include the following:

In the labor pool, drug users constitute a reserve army of easily expendable labor, filling niches in daily labor markets, construction, environmental clean-up and other areas of needed but poorly remunerated and socially devalued toil. In need of immediate cash, they are willing to take jobs with minimal wages and few worker protections. As Alysse Waterston (1993:241) pointed out, "As a special category, addicts are politically weak and disconnected from organized labor, thereby becoming a source of cheap, easily expendable labor." The existence of this group drags down wages for everyone, because at each layer of the labor force employers are able to lower the wages paid to layers above it (because other workers are said to be ready and willing to take their jobs for lower wages and fewer benefits). Given their involvement in illicit activities, drug users are less likely to contact the government about labor abuses or unsafe working conditions. Moreover, common media images of drug users as people of color promote divisive racist stereotypes that help create a controlled and internally fragmented labor force, with limited class consciousness and reduced ability to challenge actions by company owners (e.g., getting legislatures to pass so-called "right to work" laws).

Beginning in the mid-1980s, the United States began outsourcing both prison construction and the operation of prisons. The first private prison contract was awarded in 1984 to Corrections Corporation of America (CCA), which remains the largest for-profit prison company in the country. Seeking locations that would not reject the presence of a prison, private prisons often selected communities hard hit by corporate flight and the globalized economy. Heavily subsidized by taxpayer money even before receiving public contracts, private companies were able to build prisons throughout the country. For every convicted individual sent to one of its prisons, the CCA or other private prison operator receives approximately $122 a day. Based on this revenue flow, the CCA reported $1.7 billion in gross income in 2011, about half from government contracts (Carlsen 2012). But this was a time of falling crime rates. The real challenge for private prisons became filling all the cells in their newly erected prisons with convicted offenders. To drum up business and coveted profits, the private prison industry turned to lobbying in order to win stiff drug and immigration policies. The CCA 2010 Annual Report straightforwardly lays out the need for criminalization by warning its investors:

> The demand for our facilities could be adversely affected by the relaxation of enforcement efforts, leniency in conviction or parole standards and sentencing practices or through the decriminalization of certain activities that are currently proscribed by our criminal laws. For instance, any changes with respect to drugs and controlled substances or illegal immigration could affect the number of persons arrested, convicted and sentenced, thereby potentially reducing demand for correctional facilities to house them (quoted in Riggs 2012).

To insure a steady stream of new prisoners, while doing little if anything to boost public safety, private prison companies over the last decade spent over $45 million lobbying law makers. Whenever new bills were introduced that increased police power to detain suspected criminals, criminalized behaviors (such as adding new drugs to those that are illegal to sell or use) or extending prison sentences, private prisons could be found making significant campaign contributions to office holders. For example, lobbyists for the private prison industry pushed for passage of "three strikes" and "truth-in-sentencing" laws across the country. Both of these types of laws adversely impact drug users. Some of the tactics employed by private prison companies, or individuals affiliated with them, to gain influence or acquire new contracts or inmate flows included: "the use of questionable financial incentives; benefitting from the 'revolving door' between public and private corrections; extensive lobbying; lavish campaign contributions; and efforts to control information" (ACLU 2011). As a result of such labors, as the ACLU (2011) points out, "the crippling cost of imprisoning increasing numbers of Americans saddles government budgets with rising debt and exacerbates the current fiscal crises confronting states across the nation."

A set of citizens that may be readily mobilized to support campaigns for new laws or new prisons are prison employees. Prison guard unions have a strong vested economic interest in keeping people incarcerated in high numbers. In 2008, the California Correctional Peace Officers Association, for example, spent $1 million to defeat a measure that would have reduced sentences and parole times for nonviolent drug offenders while emphasizing drug treatment over imprisonment (Fang 2012). Additionally, police departments throughout the country have become dependent on federal drug war grants to fully finance their budget. To keep this money flowing, police unions see it in their best interests to lobby against drug legalization. For example, the successful campaign in 2010 against Proposition 19 in California, a ballot measure to legalize marihuana, was coordinated by a police-union lobbyist. These efforts helped insure that the police department would collect tens of millions in federal marihuana-eradication grants. Federal lobbying disclosures reveal that other police union lobbyists around the country also pushed for stiffer penalties for marihuana-related crimes. Prisoners arrested on drug charges wind up as part of an incarcerated labor pool for private corporations (e.g., in assembly) for very low wages.

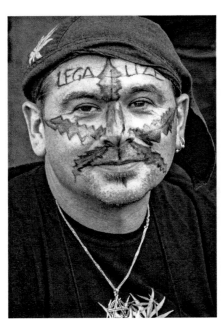

Cannabis Legalization marcher

Once behind bars, in private or public prisons, drug users become available to corporate employers who seek to profit from the super-exploitation of an incarcerated and disenfranchised workforce. They are barred from unionizing and from striking for higher wages, are silenced from protesting working conditions, and are paid bargain-basement salaries (Chien et al. 2000). Rather than the employer, the state pays the cost of sustaining this work force (e.g., food, clothes, medical care, shelter, health insurance, paid sick days or vacation time). In this system, prison guards provide unpaid (by the corporations) muscle to control the prison labor force. Prison factories, where inmates are contracted out to major corporations, operate as multibillion-dollar industries throughout the state and federal prison systems. In the agricultural sector, prison labor has become a critical labor source. In a particularly noteworthy re-writing of the rationale for the prison-industrial complex, it has been justified on the grounds that it provides inmates an opportunity to build their skills and improve their chances of post-incarceration employment.

In recent years, civil asset forfeiture laws have been passed that empower the seizures of private property even without charging anyone with violation of a law, and hence without having to prove illegal behavior beyond a reasonable doubt. Seized property, such as fast boats used to smuggle illegal drugs, is presumed to be illicitly gained or illicitly used, and can be confiscated by a police department or other government body based solely on hearsay evidence, such as a tip supplied by a government informant who stands to gain up to 25 percent of the forfeited assets. The same applies to a drug user's car or any other assets. Even medical marihuana dispensaries in California have been raided, their assets seized (e.g., ATM machines) and liquidated for cash flow to law enforcement. Confiscation may occur without an arrest because it is defined legally as an arrest of property, rather than an arrest of a person, and the necessity of proving a party guilty is not required. Numerous police, sheriff, and related law-enforcement departments around the country have embraced forfeiture laws to significantly boost their departmental budgets and budget-related perks. A study involving 90 interviews with law-enforcement officials, prosecutors, and forfeiture attorneys around the nation (Burnett 2008) suggested that police agencies that reported they were seizing property or drug money to help finance the War on Drugs appeared to be mainly doing so to help increase their own departmental budgets. Also, existing evidence shows that some officers use their badge to take cash from drivers stopped on the road for alleged drug-related suspicions without any evidence. Confiscation laws have turned the War on Drugs into a War for Funding by police and other law enforcement departments with a possibility of collapse of public oversight of these institutions.

Through various drug-money-laundering schemes—from those impli- cating banks to those involving the purchase of items (e.g., jewels or other durable goods) that are then sold to acquire "clean" money—the profits made from drug purchases help fund various sectors of the formal economy. As part of this hidden world of finance, global banking institutions like Bank of America, JP Morgan Chase & Co, Citigroup, and Wachovia among numer- ous others avoid compliance with American anti-money laundering policies. In 2010, for example, Wachovia (now Wells Fargo) orchestrated a "deferred prosecution" agreement with the US government and agreed to pay a $160 million fine following exposure of the bank's heavy involvement (to the tune of $378.4 billion over several years) in a massive money-laundering scheme. Not a single banker involved in the illegal operation was prosecuted for playing a key role in the illicit drug trade even though money laundering is absolutely vital to this global underground business. Similarly, in 2012, the US Senate Committee on Homeland Security and Governmental Af- fairs released a detailed report itemizing a catalog of "criminal" behavior by London-based HSBC Bank, a company with a long history of citations for its weak anti–money-laundering policies. The list of offenses committed by HSBC—a corporation that boasts on its website of having a firm "com- mitment to complying with the spirit and letter of all laws and regulations wherever we conduct our business"—includes washing over $881 billion for the Mexican Sinaloa Drug Cartel and for the Norte del Valle Drug Cartel in Colombia. Again, the US Department of Justice decided to cut a deal with HSBC involving a record $1.9 billion fine, which amounts to only a tiny share of the bank's annual profits of $22 billion. No company officials directly involved in illegal activities were required to spend a moment behind bars. According to Assistant US Attorney General Lanny Bauer:

> Had the U.S. authorities decided to press criminal charges, HSBC would almost certainly have lost its banking license in the U.S., the future of the institution would have been under threat and the entire banking system would have been destabilized (Murphy 2013).

Meanwhile, small-time drug dealers and drug users routinely go to prison for long sentences, the communities they come from are destabilized, and the issue of why the poor are punished but the wealthy are not disappears from public discussion.

Moreover, purchases made to facilitate drug transport (from airline tickets, to commodities used to hide drugs in, to fast boats) adds additional input to the formal economy. Luxury expenditures by the kingpins of the drug trade, individuals who may live lavish lifestyles rich in material possessions, add further cash inflow to the formal economy. The ultimate importance of drug money in the formal economy was suggested in 2009 when Antonio Maria Costa, then head of the UN Office on Drugs and Crime Drugs, reported that billions of drug dollars were used to keep the financial system afloat at the height of the global economic crisis. Claimed Costa

> In many instances, the money from drugs was the only liquid investment capital. In the second half of 2008, liquidity was the banking system's main problem and hence liquid capital became an important factor.... Inter-bank loans were funded by money that originated from the drugs trade and other illegal activities.... There were signs that some banks were rescued that way.... That was the moment ... when the system was basically paralysed because of the unwillingness of banks to lend money to one another (Syal 2009).

Even legal drug profits are impacted by the purchases of drug abusers, as people with an alcohol dependency or addiction are an important source of revenue for the alcohol industry (as are illegal drinkers like underage youth). In a report entitled "The Commercial Value of Underage and Pathological Drinking to the Alcohol Industry," the Columbia University's Center on Addiction and Substance Abuse (2006) estimated that, at a minimum, pathological drinkers and underage drinkers accounted for approximately 38 percent of alcohol-industry sales, which amounts to $50 billion, an amount that calls into question the sincerity of the frequent industry "drink responsibly" pronouncements in their advertisements and webpages.

At the bottom of the economic structure of society, drug users, through their involvement in burglaries, break-ins, muggings, and shop-lifting, and the sale of ill-gotten goods in the discounted informal economy (e.g., street sales of stolen items, sales to small stores of shop-lifted items, sale of frozen meat taken from supermarkets to small restaurants), promote a kind of trickle-down economics and a degree of wealth redistribution. Goods reach the poor, in part, because some drug users are always on the prowl for salable items that can be converted rapidly into drug money. Indeed, some have speculated that were it not for this underground redistribution of wealth the material quality of the lives of the poor would be even below current abysmal levels, although, of course, they too are subject to being stripped of their material possessions as drugs and goods flow through the street economy.

Another theme of this book is that the world of drug use, real or imagined, or some blending of the two has become a reservoir of culturally salient images, ideas, and settings harvested as a source of entertainment for everyone else. Diverse entertainment venues offer viewers and readers vicarious escape into murky, drug-driven domains of fast-paced adventure, intrigue, human suffering, comedic relief, conflict and intense aggression. Books, movies, videos, video games, music, and television dramas that feature drug users provide actors, writers, producers, directors, production company CEOs, game designers, and a host of others not only with a means of livelihood but in some cases considerable wealth. Filmmaker Matthew Cooke has even directed a how-to documentary entitled "How to Make Money Selling Drugs." While the ultimate—if not at first evident—purpose of the film is to call into question stereotypical depictions of drug users and to point out the reasons why demonization tactics are counterproductive, it is part of an educational industry that also feeds on the world of drug users.

Further, we argue in this book that the drug trade and international drug tracking is used to front initiatives designed to achieve national geo-political and geo-economic goals (Boville 2004) in cases in which direct action would be illegal or embarrassing, or would not be popular with voters. Attacking drug use can be a convenient cover for the achievement of objectives that have nothing to do with drugs, such as transferring military technology to another country to combat the drug trade (armaments that are then used to suppress social unrest and keep a "friendly" government in power). Claims of government involvement in drug trafficking were used to accuse the Chavez regime in Venezuela and the Castro Regime in Cuba of engaging in illicit drug activities, depicting these governments of illegal and immoral behavior, often with little or limited evidence, while ignoring blatant violations by friendly governments. Attacking drug producers and distributors has provided cover for other geopolitical stratagems as well. In the mid-1970s, for example, the country of Burma was the recipient of US State Department International Narcotics Control funding ostensibly to eliminate narcotics production. House Select Committee on Narcotics investigators, however, found "convincing evidence that [the] ... antinarcotics campaign is a form of economic warfare aimed at subjugation of ... Minority Peoples (U.S. Congress 1977:225). In short, drugs often have served as a Trojan Horse for the accomplishment of other aspirations. Exploiting drug use and production in the service of advancing international power is an example of what Chomsky (1988:169) has referred to as "the reality that must be effaced."

Targeting drug users as prime disruptors of urban social harmony caus-ing our streets and homes to feel unsafe, our sense of community to be a pale reflection of earlier times, and our inner cities to become eyesores that should be avoided by suburbanites, moreover, helps to render less visible structural factors that have driven urban transformation, such as the role the transnational globalization of capital has played in robbing cities of jobs with descent salaries. For example, hidden by efforts to indict drug users as the ultimate cause of multiple social problems are factory closings and their shift from right to unionize to "right-to-work" states, the further movement of production out of US cities to less expensive, less safety-focused overseas locations, rampant buy-outs and mergers that eliminate jobs and the controls imposed by competition, downsizing of a skilled and better paid work force, increasing employment of American workers in low-paying and part time jobs with limited benefits, shrinking of corporate public giving, and widening gaps between the salaries and life styles of CEOs and their employees. It is of note that when adjusted for inflation, the hourly wages of Wal-Mart employees' real salaries and standard of living have decreased steadily over time while the Walton family's wealth has increased to more than $100 billion, making them one of the wealthiest families in the United States (Wal-Mart Watch 2012).

More generally, drug users are a convenient scapegoat when things of various sorts go wrong or even when other threats to society emerge (e.g., efforts begun by the federal government in 2002 with advertisements during the Superbowl to link drug users and terrorism). Suggestions that a com-paratively high rate of drug use among the poor may, in part, be a response to structurally imposed hyperghettoization, structural violence, and social suffering caused by the detachment of capital from social responsibility to society is dismissed as "class warfare" (Singer 2008).

Even in death, drug users are useful. Cadavers used in medical-school training and in certain kinds of research are procured through established state systems from the pool of bodies of deceased individuals who are not claimed by family members or otherwise provided with means of burial. Drug users, under current social conditions, often die poor and they die often (i.e., have a high mortality rate). We have been struck in our own research by the number of deaths in our samples of drug-using study participants. Their bodies, however, provide material for the gross anatomy lessons of doctors in training, doctors who primarily will be providing their services to people—whatever their consumption patterns—not deemed by society to be drug abusers.

Given all the uses of the useless made possible by the Othering of drug users, the question must be raised: if drug user Others did not exist, would we have to invent them? Indeed, isn't this just what has happened? Based on many years of working with active, not-in-treatment consumers of mind-altering drugs, as well as being steady observers of the imagery of and attitudes about these individuals in the various cultural venues examined in this book (and the consequences of these on people's lives), our objective is to fracture imagined conception of drug users. Drug users, after all, are not really a distinct population or group of different people from us; they are our friends, relatives, colleagues, neighbors, our police officers and other first responders, our sports heroes, our warriors, our entertainers, our students, and our children.

REFERENCES

Abel, Ernest. 1999. "Was the Fetal Alcohol Syndrome Recognized by the Greeks and Romans?" *Alcohol and Alcoholism* 34(6):868–872.

―――. 2001. "Gin Lane: Did Hogarth Know About Fetal Alcohol Syndrome?" *Alcohol and Alcoholism* 36(2):131–134.

Abramson, Hilary.1998. "Big Alcohol's Smokescreen." *Newsletter of the Marin Institute for the Prevention of Alcohol & Other Drug Problems* 13:1.

ACLU. 2011, "Banking on Bondage: Private Prisons and Mass Incarceration." Available online at: http://www.aclu.org/prisoners-rights/banking-bondage-private-prisons-and-mass-incarceration.

Addams, Jane.1911. *Twenty Years at Hull-House.* New York: MacMillan.

Adrian, Bonnie. 2003. *Framing the Bride: Globalizing Beauty and Romance in Taiwan's Bridal Industry.* Berkeley: University of California Press.

Agar, Michael. 1973. *Ripping and Running: A Formal Ethnography of Urban Heroin Addicts.* New York: Academic Press.

―――. 1977. "Ethnography on the Street and in the Joint." In R. S. Weppner, ed., *Street Ethnography: Selected Studies of Crime and Drug Use in Natural Settings,* pp.143–156. Beverly Hills: Sage.

Aiken, Kristina. 2012. "Victorian Women on Drugs, Part 2: Female Writers." *Points: The Blog of the Alcohol and Drugs History Society.* Available on line at: http://pointsadhsblog.wordpress.com/2012/04/11/victorian-women-on-drugs-part-2-female-writers/.

Alcindor, Yamiche. 2012. "States Consider Drug Testing Welfare Recipients." *USA Today.* Available online at: http://usatoday30.usatoday.com/news/nation/story/2012-02-17/welfare-food-stamps-drug-testing-laws/53306804/1.

Alexander, Michelle. 2012. *The New Jim Crow: Mass Incarceration in the Age of Colorblindness.* Reprint Edition. New York: New Press.

Anderson, Margaret, and Patricia Collins, eds. 2012. *Race, Class, & Gender: An Anthology.* Independence, KY: Centage Learning.

Anonymous. 1845? *The Temperance Movement.* The University of London: Goldsmith's Library. http://find.galegroup.com/mome/infomark.do?&contentSet=MOMEArticles&type=multipage&tabID=T001&prodId=MOME&docId=U106531100&source=gale&userGroupName=miami_richter&version=1.0&docLevel=FASCIMILE.

Anselmi, William, and Kosta Gouliamos. 1998. *Elusive Margins: Consuming Media, Ethnicity, and Culture.* Toronto, Canada: Guernica

Anslinger, Harry. 1937. "The Need for Narcotics Education." *National Broadcasting Network, Anslinger Papers,* Box 1, File 7. Pennsylvania State University, Pennsylvania Historical Collections and Labor Archives, Pattee Library.

―――. 1937. "Statement of H. J. Anslinger to the U.S. Congress." Available online at: http://www.druglibrary.org/schaffer/hemp/taxact/anslng1.htm. Accessed June 14, 2013.

Anslinger, Harry, and Courtney Ryley Cooper. 1937. "Marijuana: Assassin of Youth." *The American Magazine. Anslinger Papers,* Box 1, File 11. Pennsylvania State University, Pennsylvania Historical Collections and Labor Archives, Pattee Library.

The Social Value of Drug Addicts: The Uses of the Useless, by Merrill Singer and J. Bryan Page, 219–242.

Anytown Housing Authority. 2000. "One Strike and You're Out Policy." Available online at: www.wahaonline.org/One_Strike_And_You_re_Out_Policy.docShare.

Armentano, Paul. 2010. "Incarceration Nation—Marijuana Arrests For Year 2009 Near Record High." Available online at: http://blog.norml.org/2010/09/15/incarceration-nation-marijuana-arrests-for-year-2009-near-record-high/.

Arsenault, Chris. 2012. "Mexican Official: CIA 'Manages' Drug Trade." Al Jazeera. Available online at: http://www.aljazeera.com/indepth/features/2012/07/2012721152715628181.html.

Ascherson, Neal. 2008. "Introduction." In Ryszard Kapuściński,. The Other. London: Verso.

Baer, Hans, Merrill Singer, and Ida Susser. 2013. Medical Anthropology and the World System: A Critical Perspective. Third Edition. New York City: Bergin and Garvey.

Baker, Frank, and Frank Isaacs. 1973. "Attitudes of Community Caregivers Toward Drug Users." The International Journal of the Addictions 8(2): 243–252.

Ball, Philip. 2006. The Devil's Doctor: Paracelsus and the World of Renaissance Magic and Science. New York: Farrar, Straus and Giroux.

Bandstra, Emmalee, Connie Morrow, Anthony James, Veronica Accornero, and Peter Fried. 2001. "Longitudinal Investigation of Task Persistence and Sustained Attention in Children with Prenatal Cocaine Exposure." Neurotoxicology and Teratology 23:545–559.

Bass, L. and Kane-Williams, E. 1993. "Stereotype or Reality: Another Look at Alcohol and Drug Use among African American Children." Public Health Reports 108 (Supplement 1): 78–84.

Baudelaire, Charles. 1971 [1857]. The Flowers of Evil. New York: The Heritage Press.

————. 2004 [1885]. The Poem of Hashish. New York: Kessinger Publishing Company.

Becker, Howard. 1953. "Becoming a Marihuana User." American Journal of Sociology. 59:235–242.

————. 1955. "Marihuana Use and Social Control," Social Problems 3:35–44.

————. 1963. Outsiders: Studies in the Sociology of Deviance. New York: The Free Press.

Behr, Edward. 2011. Prohibition: Thirteen Years That Changed the World. New York: Arcade Publishing

Benavidez, Edward. 2013. Getting High: The Effects of Drugs. Bloomington, IN: Xlibris Corporation.

Benet, Sula. 1975. "Early Diffusion and Folk Uses of Hemp." In Vera Rubin, ed. Cannabis and Culture, 39–50. The Hague: Mouton.

Bennett, Linda and Stephen Wolin. 1990. "Family Culture and Alcohol Transmission." In Lorraine Collins, Kenneth Leonard, and John Searles, eds, Alcohol and the Family: Research and Clinical Perspectives, 194–219. New York: The Guilford Press.

Bepko, Claudia 1991. "Introduction." In Claudia Bepko, ed. Feminism and Addiction,, 1–6. Binghamton, NY: The Haworth Press.

Besharov, Douglas. 1989. "Crack Babies: The Worst Threat Is Mom Herself." Washington Post, 1, August 6.

Bingswanger, Ingrid. 2010. "Chronic Medical Disease among Jail and Prison Inmates." Corrections.com. Available on line at: http://www.corrections.com/news/article/26014-chronic-medical-diseases-among-jail-and-prison-inmates.

Blackman, Shane. 2004. Chilling Out: The Cultural Politics of Substance Consumption, Youth and Drug Policy. Maidenhead: Open University Press.

————. 2010. "Drug War Politics: Governing Culture through Prohibition, Intoxicants as Customary Practice and the Challenge of Drug Normalization." Sociology Compass 4(10): 841–855.

Blake, John. 2012. "Return of the 'Welfare Queen,'" *CNN Politics.* Available online at: http://www.cnn.com/2012/01/23/politics/weflare-queen/index.html.

Blumenson, E., and E. Nilsen. 1998. "Policing for Profit: The Drug War's Hidden Economic Agenda." *University of Chicago Law Review* 65:35–114.

Boardman, Jason, Brian Finch, Christopher Ellison, David Williams, and James Jackson. 2001. "Neighborhood Disadvantage, Stress, and Drug Use among Adults." *Journal of Health and Social Behavior* 42:151–165.

Boeri, Miriam W., C. E. Sterk, M. Bahora, and K. Elifson. 2008. "Poly-drug use among ecstasy users: Separate, synergistic, and indiscriminate patterns." *Journal of Drug Issues* 38 (2):517–541.

Bonnie, Richard, and Charles Whitebread. 1970. "The Forbidden Fruit and the Tree of Knowledge: An Inquiry into the Legal History of American Marijuana Prohibition." *Virginia Law Review* 56(6): 971–1203.

Booth, Martin. 2003. *Cannabis: A History.* New York: Thomas Dunne Books, St. Martin's Press.

Bosmajian, Haig. 1983. *The Language of Oppression.* Lanham, MD: University Press of America.

Bourgois, Philippe. 1997. "Overachievement in the Underground Economy: The Life Story of a Puerto Rican Stick-up Artist in East Harlem." *Free Inquiry in Creative Sociology* 25(1):23–32.

———.1998. "Just Another Night in a Shooting Gallery." *Theory, Culture and Society* 15(2): 37–66.

———. 2003a. "Disciplining Addictions: The Bio-politics of Methadone and Heroin in the United States." *Culture, Medicine, and Psychiatry* 24(2): 165–195.

———. 2003b. In *Search of Respect: Selling Crack in El Barrio.* 2nd ed. Cambridge: Cambridge University Press.

Bovard, James. 1999. "Prison Sentences of the Politically Connected: Justice Has a Double Standard." *Playboy.* Online at: http://www.jimbovard.com/Bovard_Playboy_1997_Prison_Sentences_of_Politically_Connected.htm. Accessed June 11, 2013.

Bovard, James. 2008. "McCain's Forgotten Drug Fix." Online at: http://jimbovard.com/blog/2008/02/23/mccains-forgotten-drug-fix/. Accessed June 11, 2013

Boville, Belan. 2004. *The Cocaine War in Context: Drugs and Politics.* New York: Algora Publishing.

Boyd, Susan C. 2008. *Hooked: Drug War Films in Britain, Canada, and the United States.* New York: Routledge.

Brissett-Chapman, S. 1998. "Homeless African-American Women and Their Families: Coping with Depression, Drugs, and Trauma." In C. Wetherington and A. Roman, eds., 503–516. *Drug Addiction Research and the Health of Women.* Rockville, MD: National Institutes of Health, US Department of Health and Human Services.

Brook, J., Cohen, P., and Brook, E. 1998. "Longitudinal Study of Co-occurring Psychiatric Disorders and Substance Use." *Journal of the American Academy of Child and Adolescent Psychiatry* 37(3): 322–330.

Brown, Claude. 1965. *Manchild in the Promised Land.* New York: Touchstone.

Buchanan, David, Susan Shaw, Amy Ford, and Merrill Singer. 2003. "Empirical Science Meets Moral Panic: An Analysis of the Politics of Needle Exchange." *Journal of Public Health Policy* 24(3/4): 427–444.

Bunce, R. 1979. "The political economy of California's wine industry. Manuscript prepared for the International Study of Alcohol Control Experiences Project." Addiction

Research Foundation, Toronto.Burchard, R. 1992. "Coca Chewing and Diet." *Current Anthropology* 33:1–24.

Burchard, Roderick 1976. "Myths of the Sacred Leaf: Ecological Perspective on Coca and Peasant Biocultural Adaptation in Peru." PhD dissertation, Indiana University.

Burnett, John. 2008. "Sheriff under Scrutiny over Drug Money Spending." National Public Radio. Available online at: http://www.npr.org/templates/story/story.php?storyId=91638378.

Burns, Ken and Lynn Novick. 2011. *Prohibition*.

Burroughs, William. 1953. *Junkie*. New York: Ace Books.

———. 1959. *Naked Lunch*. New York: Grove Press.

———. 1961. *The Soft Machine*. Paris: Olympia Press.

———.1962. *The Ticket that Exploded*. Paris: Olympia Press.

———. 1964. *Nova Express*. New York: Grove Press.

Burston, B., D. Jones, and P. Roberson-Saunders. 1995. "Drug Use and African Americans: Myth versus Reality." *Journal of Alcohol and Drug Education* 40:19–39.

Burton, Robert. 2000 [1621]. *The Anatomy of Melancholy*. Oxford, England: Clarendon Press; New York: Oxford University Press.

Campbell, Nancy. 2000. *Using Women: Gender, Drug Policy, and Social Justice*. New York: Routledge.

Carlsen, Laura. 2012. "How Private Prisons Profit from the Criminalization of Immigrants." *Counterpunch*, December 28–30. Available online at: http://www.counterpunch.org/2012/12/12/how-private-prisons-profit-from-the-criminalization-of-immigrants/.

Carroll, Rebecca. 2004. "Under the Influence: Harry Anslinger's Role in Shaping America's Drug Policy." In Jonathon Erlen and Joseph Spillane, eds. *Federal Drug Control: The Evolution of Policy and Practice*, 61. Binghamton, NY: Pharmaceutical Products Press.

Carter, Henry. 1933. *The English Temperance Movement: A Study in Objectives*. London: The Epworth Press.

Carter, William. 1977. "Ritual, the Aymara, and the Role of Alcohol in Human Society." In B. M. DuToit, ed. *Drugs, Rituals, and Altered States of Consciousness*, 101–110. Rotterdam: Balkema.

Carter, William, and Mauricio P. Mamani. 1986. *Coca en Bolivia*. La Paz: Editorial Juventud.

Carter, William, Wilmer Coggins, and Paul Doughty, eds. 1980. *Cannabis in Costa Rica*. Philadelphia: ISHI Press.

Carter, William, J. Bryan Page, Paul Doughty, and Wilmer Coggins. 1980. "Marijuana in Costa Rica." In William Carter, Paul Doughty, and Wilmer Coggins, eds. *Cannabis in Costa Rica*. 12–40. Philadelphia: ISHI Press.

Chambliss, William. 1994. "Don't Confuse me with Facts: Clinton 'Just Says No.'" *New Left Review* (March/April). Online at: http://newleftreview.org/I/204/william-j-chambliss-don-t-confuse-me-with-facts-clinton-just-says-no.

Chen, C., M. Dufour, and H. Yi. 2003. "Alcohol Consumption Among Young Adults Ages 18–24 in the United States: Results From the 2001-2002 NESARC Survey." *Alcohol: Research and Health* 28(4): 269–280.

Chesney-Lind, Meda, and Lisa Pakso. 2004. *The Female Offender*. Thousand Oaks, CA: Sage.

Chien, Arnold, Margaret Connors, and Kenneth Fox. 2000. "The Drug War in Perspective." In Jim Kim, Joyce Millen, Alec Irwin, and John Gershman. 293–327. Monroe, ME: Common Courage Press.

Chiricos, T. 1996. "Moral Panics as Ideology: Drugs, Violence, Race and Punishment in

America." In M. Lynch and E. Britt Patterson, eds. *Race with Prejudice: Race and Justice in America.* 19–48. New York: Harrow and Heston.

Chomsky, Noam. 1988. *The Culture of Terrorism.* Boston: South End Press.

Christie, Agatha. 1924. *Poirot Investigates.* New York: Penguin Group.

Clayton, Richard R., and Harwin L. Voss. 1981. *Young Men and Drugs in Manhattan: A Causal Analysis.* Monogaph #39. Rockville, MD: NIDA.

Cloward, Richard, and Lloyd Ohlin. 1960. *Delinquency and Opportunity: A Theory of Delinquent Gangs.* New York: The Free Press of Glencoe.

CNN.com. 2005. "New Orleans Mayor Lashes Out at Feds." Available at http://www.cnn.com/2005/US/09/02/katrina.nagin/index.html.

Cohen, Albert. 1955. *Delinquent Boys: The Culture of the Gang.* New York: The Free Press of Glencoe.

Cohen, Stanley. 1972. *Folk Devils and Moral Panics.* London: MacGibbon and Kee Ltd.

Columbia University's Center on Addiction and Substance Abuse. 2006. *The Commercial Value of Underage and Pathological Drinking to the Alcohol Industry.* New York: CASA.

Community Epidemiology Work Group. 2011. *Epidemiologic Trends in Drug Abuse,* Volume II. Bethesda, MD: National Institute on Drug Abuse.

Cook, Christopher C.H. 2006. *Alcohol, Addiction, and Christian Ethics.* Cambridge: Cambridge University Press.

Cooke, Janet. 1980. "Jimmy's World." *Washington Post,* September 28, A1. http://www.uncp.edu/home/canada/work/markport/lit/litjour/spg2002/cooke.htm.

Coomber, Ross, ed. 1994. *Drugs and Drug Use in Society: A Critical Reader.* Dartford, UK: Greenwich University Press.

Coomber, Ross, Craig Morris, and Laura Dunn. 2000. "How the Media Do Drugs: Quality Control and the Reporting of Drug Issues in the UK Print Media." *International Journal of Drug Policy* 11:217–225.

Correction Association of New York. 2011. Treatment Behind Bars: Substance Abuse Treatment in New York State Prisons, 2007-2010. New York: Correctional Association of New York.

Courtwright, David. 2001. *Forces of Habit: Drugs and the Making of the Modern World.* Cambridge, MA: Harvard University Press.

Courtwright, David, Joseph, Herman and Des Jarlais, Don. 1989. *Addicts who survived: An oral history of narcotic use in American, 1923-1965.* Knoxville, TN: University of Tennessee Press.

Covington, J. 1997. "The Social Construction of the Minority Drug Problem." *Social Justice* 24:117–147.

Cressey, Donald R. 1962. "Role Theory, Differential Association, and Compulsive Crimes," In Arnold M. Rose, ed. *Human Behavior and Social Processes, An Interactionist Approach.* Boston: Houghton Mifflin Co. pp. 444–467.

Crowley, Aleister. 1922. *Diary of a Drug Fiend.* New York: Ordo Templi Orientis.

CSAP/ICAP Joint Working Group on Terminology. 1998. "Working Papers." Online at: http://www.icap.org/portals/0/download/all_pdfs/Other_Publications/CSAP_ICAP_Terminology.pdf.

Dallas Morning News. 2009. Editorial: Drug Users Share the Blame in officer's death. Available at http://nl.newsbank.com/nl-search/we/Archives?p_product=DM&p_theme=dm&p_action=search&p_maxdocs=200&s_hidethis=no&p_field_label-0=Author&p_field_label-1=title&p_bool_label-1=AND&p_text_label-1=Drug%20Users%20Share%20Blame%20in%20Officer's%20Death&p_field_label-2=

Section&p_bool_label-2=AND&s_dispstring=headline(Drug%20Users%20Share
%20Blame%20in%20Officer's%20Death)%20AND%20date(01/10/2008%20to%20
01/10/2009)&p_field_date-0=YMD_date&p_params_date-0=date:B,E&p_text_
date-0=01/10/2008%20to%2001/10/2009)&p_perpage=10&p_sort=YMD_
date:D&xcal_useweights=no

Daly, Kathleen. 1998. "Gender, Crime, and Criminology." In *The Handbook of Crimes and Justice*, Michael Tonrey, ed., 85–108. Oxford: Oxford University Press.

Davenport-Hines, Richard. 2002. *The Pursuit of Oblivion: A Global History of Narcotics*. New York: W.W. Norton and Company.

Davidson, J. 1999. "The Drug War's Color Line: Black Leaders Shift Stances on Sentencing." *The Nation* 269(8): 42–43.

Davies, Paul, Howard Iams, and Kalman Rupp. 2000. "The Effect of Welfare Reform on SSA's Disability Programs: Design of Policy Evaluation and Early Evidence." *Social Security Bulletin* 63(1): 3–11.

Davis, J. Francis. 1992. "Power of Images: Creating the Myths of Our Time." *Media and Values* 57(Winter). Available online at: http://www.medialit.org/reading-room/power-images-creating-myths-our-time. Accessed April 30, 2011.

DAWN—Drug Abuse Warning Network. 2009. "Emergency Presentations for Drug Related Problems." Available at: https://dawninfo.samhsa.gov/default.asp.

De La Rosa, Mario R., and Juan-Luis Recio Adrados, 1993. *Drug Abuse among Minority Youth: Methodological Issues and Recent Research Advances*. NIDA Monograph 130. Rockville, MD: NIDA.

de Quincey, Thomas. 1822. *Confessions of an English Opium Eater*. New York: F. M. Lupton.

DEA. 2011. *The DEA Position on Marijuana*. Washington, DC: DEA.

Diala, C., C. Muntaner, and C. Walrath. 2004. "Gender, Occupational, and Socioeconomic Correlates of Alcohol and Drug Abuse among U.S. Rural, Metropolitan, and Urban Residents." *American Journal of Drug and Alcohol Abuse* 30(2), 409–428.

Dingelstad, D., R. Gosden, B. Martin, and N. Vakas. 1996. "The Social Construction of Drug Debates." *Social Science and Medicine* 43: 1829–1838.

Dobkin de Rios, Marlene. 1970. "Banisteriopsis Used in Witchcraft and Folk Healing in Iquitos, Peru." *Economic Botany* 24(35): 296–300.

Dobkin de Rios, Marlene.1971. "Ayahuasca, the Healing Vine." *International Journal of Social Psychiatry* 17(4): 256–269.

Dobkin de Rios, Marlene.1972a. "Curing with Ayahuasca in a Peruvian Amazon Slum." In M. J. Harner, ed. *Hallucinogens and Shamanism*. New York: Oxford University Press.

Dobkin de Rios, Marlene. 1972b. *Visionary Vine: Psychedelic Healing in the Peruvian Amazon*. San Francisco: Chandler Publishing Company.

Dobkin de Rios, Marlene 2005. "Interview with Guillermo Arrevalo, a Shipibo Urban Shaman by Roger Rumrrill." *Journal of Psychoactive Drugs* 37 (2): 203–207.

Doctor, Ronald, and Nicholas Sieveking. 1973." A Comparison of Attitudes among Heroin Addicts, Policemen, Marijuana Users, and Nondrug Users about the Drug Addict." *The International Journal of the Addictions* 8(4): 691–699.

Donnelly, Taylor. 2012. "'Just One Step Away': The Mad Other on the Contemporary Stage." *Otherness: Essays and Studies* 2(2):1–28.

Douglas, Susan, and Meredith Michaels. 2004. *The Mommy Myth: The Idealization of Motherhood and How It Has Undermined All Women*. New York: Free Press.

Downes, D. 1977. "The Drug Addict as Folk Devil." In P. Rock, eds. *Drugs and Politics*. New Brunswick, NJ: Transaction Books.

Drake, St. C., and Horace Cayton. 1970. *Black Metropolis: A Study of Negro Life in a Northern City*, Vol. 2. New York: Harcourt, Brace and World.

Dreher, M. C. 1982. *Working Men and Ganja: Marihuana Use in Rural Jamaica.* Philadelphia: ISHI Press.

Drug Enforcement Administration. 2009. "Think Drug Use Doesn't Hurt anyone? Think Twice." Available at http://www.justthinktwice.com/costs/.

Drug Enforcement Agency. 2013. "Appropriations Table." Available at http://www.justice.gov/dea/about/history/staffing.shtml.

Drug Policy Alliance. 2002. "Police, Drugs and Corruption: A Review of Recent Drug-War Related Scandals in Five States and Puerto Rico." Available online at: https://www.google.com/search?sourceid=navclient&aq=&oq=Police%2C+Drugs+and+Corruption%3A+A+Review+of++Recent+Drug-War+related+Scandals+in+Five+States+and+Puerto+&ie=UTF-8&rlz=1T4GGLL_enUS400US400&q=Police%2C+Drugs+and+Corruption%3A+A+Review+of++Recent+Drug-War+related+Scandals+in+Five+States+and+Puerto+&gs_l=hp....0.0.0.1765..........0.

Drug Policy Alliance Network. 2005. "Drug Users Demonized by Hurricane Coverage." Available at http://www.drugpolicy.org/news/090905hurricane.cfm.

Dudley, Robert. 2002. "Fermenting Fruit and the Historical Ecology of Ethanol Ingestion: Is Alcoholism in Modern Humans an Evolutionary Hangover?" *Addiction* 97:381–388.

Dugsdale, D. 2011. "Delirium Tremens. Medline Plus." Available online at: http://www.nlm.nih.gov/medlineplus/ency/article/000766.htm.

DuPont, Robert. 1974. "The Evolving Federal Substance Abuse Organization." *The American Journal of Drug and Alcohol Abuse* 1(1):1–9.

Dushay, Robert, Merrill Singer, Margaret Weeks, Lucy Rohena, and Richard Gruber. 2001. "Lowering HIV Risk Among Ethnic Minority Drug Users: Comparing Culturally Targeted Intervention to a Standard Intervention." *American Journal of Drug and Alcohol Abuse* 27(3): 504–524.

Edelman, Murray. 1988. *Constructing the Political Spectacle.* Chicago: University of Chicago.

Edgar Allan Poe Society. 2009. "Edgar Allan Poe, Drugs and Alcohol." Available on line at: http://www.eapoe.org/geninfo/poealchl.htm.

Ehrman, Mark. 1995. "Heroin Chic." *Playboy* 42:5.

Eisenhower, Dwight. 1953. "The Change for Peace" speech. Available online at: http://www.edchange.org/multicultural/speeches/ike_chance_for_peace.html.

Eisenstein, Elizabeth. 1980. *The Printing Press as an Agent of Change.* Cambridge: Cambridge University Press.

Elliot, Deni. 2011. "Ethical Responsibilities and the Power of Pictures." In Susan Ross and Park Lestor, eds. *Images that Injure: Pictorial Stereotypes in the Media,* 9–19. Santa Barbara: Praeger.

Engels, Friedrich. 1845 and 1972 [2001]. *The Condition of the Working Class in England.* London: Electric Books.

Ensminger, M., J. Anthony, and J. McCord. 1997. "The Inner City and Drug Use: Initial Findings from an Epidemiological Study." *Drug and Alcohol Dependence* 48:175–184.

Epstein, Jennifer, and Gilbert Botvin, 2002. "The Moderating Role of Risk-Taking Tendency and Refusal Assertiveness on Social Influences in Alcohol Use among Inner-City Adolescents." *Journal of Studies on Alcohol* 63 (4): 456–459.

Erwin, William E., Dianne B. Williams, and William A. Speir. 1998. "Delirium Tremens." *Southern Medical Journal* 91(5): 425–532.

Evans-Pritchard, Edward. 1940. *The Nuer, a Description of the Modes of Livelihood and Political Institutions of a Nilotic People.* Oxford: Clarendon Press.

Ezard, John. 2000. "The Story of Dr Jekyll, Mr Hyde and Fanny, the Angry Wife Who Burned the First Draft." *The Guardian.* Available on line at http://www.guardian.co.uk/uk/2000/oct/25/books.booksnews.

Fang, Lee. 2012. "The Top Five Special Interest Groups Lobbying to Keep Marijuana Illegal." *Republic Report,* April 20. Available online at: http://www.republicreport.org/2012/marijuana-lobby-illegal/.

Feiling, Tom. 2010. *Cocaine Nation: How The White Trade Took Over The World.* New York: Pegasus.

Feldman, Harvey, and Michael Aldrich. 1990. "The role of ethnography in substance abuse research and public policy: Historical precedent and future prospects." In Elizabeth Lambert, ed., *The Collection and interpretation of Data from Hidden Populations.* Pp. 13–30. National Institute on Drug Abuse Research.

Fine, Michelle. 1994. "Working the Hyphens: Reinvention Self and Other in Qualitative Research." In *Handbook of Qualitative Research.* Norman Denzin and Yvonna Lincoln, eds, pp. 70-82. Thousand Oaks, CA: Sage Publications.

FitzGerald, Edward. 2011. *The Rubáiyát of Omar Khayyám.* New York: Dover Publications.

Fitzgerald, F. Scott. 1993. The Great Gatsby. Ware, Herts, UK: Wordsworth Editions.

Fleming, Alice, M. 1975. *Alcohol: The Delightful Poison.* New York: Dell Publishing Company.

Fox, Tracy Gordon. 2002. "Death at Hotel Hooker." Available online at: http://www.courant.com/news/specials/hc-2heroin.artoct21,0,5402919.story?page=1. Accessed 5/4/2011.

Fox, Tracy Gordon, and Bill Leukhardt. 2002a. "Small Town, Big-Time Heroin Use." *The Hartford Courant,* October 20. Available online at: http://www.courant.com/news/special-reports/hc-1heroin.artoct20,0,842029.story?page=1. Accessed May 1, 2011.

Fox, Tracy Gordon, and Bill Leukhardt. 2002b. "Can't Somebody Do Something?" Available online at: http://www.courant.com/news/special-reports/hc-5heroin.artoct24,0,5298485.story?page=1. Accessed May 4, 2011.

Foxcroft, Louise. 2007. *The Making of Addiction: The 'Use and Abuse' of Opium in Nineteenth-Century Britain.* Hampshire, UK: Ashgate Publishing Limited.

Freeth, Tony. 1985. "Racism on Television: Bringing the Colonies Back Home." In Phil Cohen and Carl Gardner, Carl, eds., *It Ain't Half Racist, Mum—Fighting Racism in the Media.* London: Comedia Publishing Group.

Friedman, Samuel. 1998. "The Political Economy of Drug-user Scapegoating—and the Philosophy and Politics of Resistence." *Drugs: Education and Policy* 5(1):15–32.

Fuller Crystal, Vlahova, David, Ompad, Danielle, Shah, Nina, Arria, Amelia and Strathdee, Steffanie. 2002. "High-risk behaviors associated with transition from illicit non-injection to injection drug use among adolescent and young adult drug users: a case-control study." *Drug and Alcohol Dependence* 2(1):189-198.

Furnas, Joseph C. 1965. *The Life and Times of the Late Demon Rum.* New York: G.P. Putnam's Sons.

Furst, Peter. 1972. "To Find Our Life: Peyote among the Huichol Indians in Mexico." In P. T. Furst, ed., *Flesh of the Gods,* 136–184. Prospect Heights, IL: Waveland Press.

Furst, Peter. 2006. *Rock Crystals & Peyote Dreams: Explorations in the Huichol Universe.* Salt Lake City: University of Utah Press.

Galea, S., J. Ahern, M. Tracy, and D. Vlahov. 2007. "Neighborhood Income and Income

Distribution and the Use of Cigarettes, Alcohol, and Marijuana." *American Journal of Preventive Medicine* 32(6): 195–202.

Genberg, Becky, Stephen Gange, Vivian Go, David Celentano, Kirk, Carl Gregory, and Shruti Mehta,2011. "The Effect of Neighborhood Deprivation and Residential Relocation on Long-term Injection Cessation among Injection Drug Users (IDUs) in Baltimore, Maryland." *Addiction* 106(11): 1966–1974.

Gilens, Martin. 1999. *Why Americans Hate Welfare: Race, Media and the Politics of Antipoverty Policy.* Chicago: University of Chicago Press.

Gilliam, Franklin 1999. "The 'Welfare Queen' Experiment: How Viewers React to Images of African-American Mothers on Welfare." *Nieman Reports.* Cambridge, MA: The Nieman Foundation for Journalism at Harvard University 53(2):49–52.

Gladwell, Malcolm. 2005. *Blink: The Power of Thinking without Thinking.* New York: Little, Brown, and Company.

Global Commission on Drug Policy. 2011. "Report of the Global Commission on Drug Policy." Availble on line at: globalcommissionondrugs.org

Goffman, Erving. 1963. *Stigma: Notes on the Management of Spoiled Identity.* Englewood Cliffs, NJ: Prentice-Hall.

Goldstein, P., B. Spunt, T. Miller, and P. Bellucci. 1990. "Ethnographic Field Stations." In E. Lambert, ed, *The Collection and Interpretation of Data from Hidden Populations,* Monograph 98, 80–95. Rockville, MD: National Institute on Drug Abuse Research.

Goode, Erich. 1984. *Drugs in American Society.* New York: Alfred A. Knopf.

Goodman, Jordan. 1993. *Tobacco in History: The Cultures of Dependence.* New York: Routledge.

Gordon, Diana. 1994. "Drugspeak and the Clinton Administration: A Lost Opportunity for Drug Policy Reform." *Social Justice* 21(3): 30–37.

Gossip, Michael. 1996. *Living with Drugs.* London: Ashgate Publishing Limited.

Government Accountability Office. 2012. *Growing Inmate Crowding Negatively Affects Inmates, Staff and Infrastructure.* Washington, D.C.: GAO.

Gramsci, Antonio. 1971. *Selections from the Prison Notebooks.* London: Lawrence and Wishart.

Grant, Igor, J. Atkinson, Gouaux Hampton, Ben Barth, and Wilsey Barth. 2012. "Medical Marijuana: Clearing Away the Smoke." *The Open Neurology Journal* 6:18–25.

Grau, Lauretta, T. Green, Merrill Singer, Ricky Bluthenthal, Patricia Marshall, and Robert Heimer. 2009. "Getting the Message Straight: Effects of a Brief Hepatitis Prevention Intervention among Injection Drug Users." *Harm Reduction Journal* (on-line journal) 6:36.

Green, E. 1914. "Psychoses among Negroes—A Comparative Study." *Journal of Nervous and Mental Disease* 41: 697–708.

Gregory, Steven. 1996. "Race, Rubbish, and Resistance: Empowering Difference in Community Politics." *Cultural Anthropology* 8(1): 24–48.

Grivetti, L. 1995. "Wine: The Food with Two Faces." In P. E. McGovern, S. J. Fleming, and S. J. Katz, eds, *The Origins and Ancient History of Wine,* 9–22. Luxembourg: Gordon & Breach, Publishers.

Gross, Dave. 1995. "A Brief Biography of Fitz Hugh Ludlow." Online at: http://users.lycaeum.org/~sputnik/Ludlow/THE/Biography/biography.html. Accessed June 13, 2013.

Grotenhermen, Franjo, Gero Leson, Gunter Berghaus, Olaf H. Drummer, Hans-Peter Kruger, Marie Longo, Herbert Moskowitz, Bud Perrine, Johannes G. Ramaekers, Alison Smiley, and Rob Tunbridge. 2007. "Developing Limits for Driving under Cannabis." *Addiction.* 102(12): 1910–1917.

Gusfield, Joseph. 1963. *Symbolic Crusade: Status Politics and the American Temperance Movement.* Urbana: University of Illinois Press.

Gusfield, Joseph. 1996. *Contested Meanings: The Construction of Alcohol Problems.* Madison, WI: University of Wisconsin Press.

Gustason, Kaaryn. 2012. *Cheating Welfare: Public Assistance and the Criminalization of Poverty.* New York City: New York University Press.

Halnon, Karen. 2009. "Heroin Chic, Poor Chic, and Beyond Deconstructionist Distraction." *Consumers, Commodities and Consumption* 11(1): 1–3.

Harner, Michael J. 1973a. "The Role of Hallucinogenic Plants in European Witchcraft." In Michael J. Harner, Ed. *Hallucinogens and Shamanism,* pp. 15–27. New York: Oxford University Press.

Harner, Michael J. 1973b. "The Sound of Rushing Water." In Michael J. Harner, Ed. *Hallucinogens and Shamanism,* pp. 28–27. New York: Oxford University Press.

Harner, Michael J. 1990. *The Way of the Shaman.* San Francisco: Harper & Row.

Harrington, Thomas. 2011. Statement for the Record before the Senate Caucus on International Narcotics Control. United States Senate. Online at: http://www.justice.gov/dea/pr/speeches-testimony/2012-2009/110525_ca_security_cooperation.pdf. Accessed August 8, 2013.

Hart, Carl. 2013. *High Price: A Neuroscientist's Journey of Self-Discovery That Challenges Everything You Know About Drugs and Society.* New York: HarperCollins Publishers.

Heath, Dwight. 1958. "Drinking Patterns of the Bolivian Camba." *Quarterly Journal of Studies on Alcohol* 19: 491–508.

Heath, Dwight. 1976. "Anthropological Perspectives on Alcohol: An Historical Review." In M. Everett, ed. *Cross-Cultural Approaches to the Study of Alcohol: An Interdisciplinary Approach.* The Hague, Netherlands: Mouton.

Heath, Dwight. 1991. "Continuity and Change in Drinking Patterns of the Bolivian Camba." In D. Pittman and H. White, eds, *Society, Culture, and Drinking Patterns Reexamined,* 78–84. New Brunswick, NJ: Rutgers Center of Alcohol Studies.

Heath, Dwight. 2004 Camba (Bolivia) "Drinking Patterns: Changes in Alcohol Use, Anthropology, and Research Perspectives." In *Drug Use and Cultural Contexts: Beyond the West,* ed. R. Coomber and N. South, 119–136. London: Free Association Books.

Heckel, E. A., and C. Dea Moore. 2009. "Community-Based Participatory Research: The College as the Focal Community." *Journal of Baccalaureate Social Work* 14 (1): 45–61.

Hedrick, J. 1994. *Harriet Beecher Stowe: A Life.* New York: Oxford University Press.

Helmer, John. 1983. "Blacks and Cocaine." In *Drugs and Society,* Maureen Kelleher, Bruce MacMurray, and Thomas Shapiro, eds., 14–29. Dubuque, IA: Kendall/Hunt.

Hickman, Timothy. 2009. *Heroin Chic: The Visual Culture of Narcotics Addiction.* Third Text 16(2):119–136.

Hillman, D. 2008. *The Chemical Muse: Drug Use and the Roots of Western Civilization.* New York: St. Martin's Press.

Hodgins, D., N. Ed-Guebaly, and J. Addington. 1997. "Treatment of Substance Abusers: Single or Mixed Gender Programs?" *Addiction* 92(7): 805–812.

Hopfer, Christian, Khuri, Elizabeth, Crowley, Thomas, and Hooks, Sabrina. 2002. "Adolescent heroin use: a review of the descriptive and treatment literature." *Journal of Substance Abuse Treatment* 23(3):321-237.Hopkins, Ellen. 2003. *Crank.* New York: Simon and Schuster.

Huff, Darrell. 1954. *How to Lie with Statistics.* New York: W. W. Norton.

Huffman, Michael. 2003. "Animal Self-Medication and Ethno-medicine: Exploration of Medicinal Properties of Plants." *Proceedings of the Nutritional Society* 62:371–381.

Huisenga, Sarah. 2011. "Newt Gringrich: Poor Kids Don't Work 'unless it's illegal.'" CBS News. December 1. Available online at: http://www.cbsnews.com/8301-503544_162-57335118-503544/newt-gingrich-poor-kids-dont-work-unless-its-illegal/.

Human Rights Watch. 2009. *Decades of Disparity: Drug Arrests and Race in the United States.* New York: Human Rights Watch.

Human Rights Watch. 2012. *Sex Workers at Risk: Condoms as Evidence of Prostitution in Four US Cities.* Washington: Human Rights Watch.

Hutchinson, Asa. 2002. "Narco-Terror: The International Connection Between Drugs and Terror." Speech delivered at the Heritage Foundation: Kathryn and Shelby Cullom Davis Institute for International Studies, Washington, D.C. Available online at: http://www.justice.gov/dea/pr/speeches-testimony/2002/s040202p.html. Accessed August 8, 2013.

Humphries, Drew. 1999. *Crack Mothers: Pregnancy, Drugs, and the Media.* Columbus: Ohio State University Press.

Humphries, Drew, J. Dawson, V. Cronin, P. Keating, C.Wisniewski, and J. Eichfeld. 1992. "Mothers and Children, Drugs and Crack: Reactions to Maternal Drug Dependency." In *The Criminalization of a Woman's Body.* C. Feldman, ed. New York: The Haworth Press.

Huxley, Aldous. 1932. *Brave New World.* London: Chatto and Windus.

Huxley, Aldous. 1954. *The Doors of Perception.* London: Chatto and Windus.

Iiyama, Patti, Setsuko, Nishi, and Johnson Bruce. 1976. *Drug Use and Abuse among U.S. Minorities: An Annotated Bibliography.* New York: Praeger.

Inciardi, James. 1989. Personal communication to Bryan Page.

Inciardi, James, and K. McElrath, eds, *The American Drug Scene*, 225–229. Los Angeles: Roxbury Publishing Company.

Ingram, Allan. 1998. "Samuel Taylor Coleridge, letter to John J. Morgan (1814)." *Patterns of Madness in the Eighteenth Century,* 200–224. Chicago: University of Chicago Press.

International Center for Alcohol Policies (ICAP). 2012. *Producers, Sellers, and Drinkers: Studies of Noncommercial Alcohol in Nine Countries.* Washington, D.C.: ICAP.

Izant, Eric. 2008. "Altered States of Style: The Drug-Induced Development of Jack Kerouac's Spontaneous Prose." Master's Thesis. Brigham Young University.

Jackson, Janine. 1998. "The Myth of the 'Crack Baby.'" *Fairness and Accuracy in Reporting,* October. Online at: http://www.fair.org/index.php?page=3702.

James, W., and S. Johnson. 1996. *Doin' Drugs: Patterns of African American Addiction.* Austin: University of Texas Press.

Jeffery, Roger. 1979. "Normal Rubbish: Deviant Patients in Casualty Departments." *Sociology of Health and Illness* 1(1): 90–107.

Johnson, Paul. 1978. *A Shopkeeper's Millenium: Society and Revivals in Rochester, New York, 1815–1837.* New York: Hill and Wang.

Johnston, Lloyd D., Patrick M. O'Malley, and Jerald G. Bachman,.1985. *Use of Licit and Illicit Drugs by America's High School Students 1975–1984.* Rockville, MD: DHHS Publication No. (ADM) 85-1394.

Johnston, Lloyd, Patrick O'Malley, and Jerald Bachman,. 1986. *Drug Use Among American High School Students, College Students, and Other Young Adults: National Trends through 1985.* Rockville, MD: National Institute on Drug Abuse.

Jones, Kenneth, David Smith, Christy Ulleland, and Ann Streissig. 1973. "Pattern of

Malformation in Offspring of Chronic Alcoholic Mothers." *Lancet* 1 (7815): 1267–1271.

Joyce Foundation . 2002. *Welfare to Work: What Have We Learned.* Chicago: The Joyce Foundation.

Kallen, Evelyn. 1989. *Label Me Human: Minority Rights of Stigmatized Canadians.* Toronto: University of Toronto Press.

Kandel, Denise, Gebre-Egziabher Kiros, Christine Schaffran. 2004. "Racial/Ethnic Differences in Cigarette Smoking Initiation and Progression to Daily Smoking: a Multilevel Analysis." *American Journal of Public Health* 94 (1): 128–136.

Kapuściński, Ryszard. 2008. *The Other.* London: Verso.

Kauffman, S., P. Silver,. and J. Poulin, 1997. "Gender Differences in Attitudes toward Alcohol, Tobacco, and Other Drugs." *Social Work* 42(3): 231–241.

Keller, M. 1979. "A Historical Overview of Alcohol and Alcoholism." *Cancer Research* 39: 2822–2829.

Kennedy, David, and Sue-Lin Wong. 2009. *The High Point Market Intervention Strategy.* New York City: Center for Crime Prevention and Control, John Jay College of Criminal Justice.

Kerr, Peter. 1986. "Rising Concern on Drugs Stirs Public to Activism." *New York Times,* August 10, A1, 28.

Kessler, Glenn. 2011. "Haley Barbour's Medicaid Fantasy." The Washington Post. Available online at: http://voices.washingtonpost.com/fact-checker/2011/03/haley_barbours_medicaid_fantas.html.

Kilbourne, Jean. 1990. Deadly Persuasion: "7 Myths Alcohol Advertisers Want You to Believe." *Media and Values* 54–55. Available online at: http://www.medialit.org/reading-room/deadly-persuasion-7-myths-alcohol-advertisers-want-you-believe.

Kimiya, Gary. 2000. "Writing High." Salon. August 4. Online at: http://www.salon.com/2000/08/04/drugs_11/. Accessed June 13, 2013.

King, David. 1999. *The Commissar Vanishes: The Falsification of Photographs and Art in Stalin's Russia.* Chicago: Holt.

King, Stephen. 2000. *On Writing, A Memoir of The Craft.* New York: Scribner.

Kipling, Rudyard. 2010 [1884]. "The Gate of the Hundred Sorrows." Available online at: http://en.wikisource.org/wiki/The_Gate_of_the_Hundred_Sorrows.

Kitton, Frederick. 1897. *The Novels of Charles Dickens: A Bibliography and Sketch.* London: Elliot Stock.

Kleiman, Mark, Jonathan Caukins, and Hawkens, Jonathan. 2012. "Rethinking the War on Drugs. The Saturday Essay." *Wall Street Journal.* Available on line at: http://online.wsj.com/article/SB10001424052702303425504577353754196169014.html.

Knipe, Edward. 1995. *Culture, Society, and Drugs: The Social Science Approach to Drug Use.* Prospect Heights, IL: Waveland Press.

Koester Stephen, J. Glanz, and A. Baron. 2005. "Drug Sharing among Heroin Networks: Implications for HIV and Hepatitis B and C Prevention." *AIDS and Behavior* 9(1): 27–39.

Kreiger, Nancy. 2005. *Health Disparities and the Body.* Boston: Harvard School of Public Health.

La Barre, Weston. 1975 [original 1938]. *The Peyote Cult.* Hamden, CT: Archon Books.

La Barre, Weston, D. McAllester, J. S. Slotkin, Omar Stewart, and Sol Tax. 1951. "Statement on Peyote." *Science* 114:582–583.

Labute, Neil. 2004. *Fat Pig.* New York: Faber and Faber.

Lee, J. 1989. *Thinking about Higher Order Thinking: Abstraction and Stereotype Thinking in Education.* DeKalb, IL: Social Science Research Institute: Northern Illinois University.

Leibling, A. J. 1947. "Horsefeathers Swathed in Mink." *New Yorker.* Available online at: http://www.newyorker.com/archive/1947/11/22/1947_11_22_066_TNY_ CARDS_000212206.

Lender, Mark and James Kirby. 1982. *Drinking in America.* New York: The Free Press.

Levine, Harry Gene. 1978. "The Discovery of Addictions: Changing Conceptions of Habitual Drunkenness in America." *Journal of Studies on Alcohol* 39(1): 143–174.

Li, Hui-Lin. 1974. "An Archaeological and Historical Account of Cannabis in China." *Economic Botany* 28(4):437–448.

Lindesmith, Alfred. 1940. "Dope Fiend Mythology." *Journal of Criminal Law and Criminology* 31(2): 199–208.

Link, B., E. Struening, M. Rahav, J. Phelan, and L. Nuttbrock. 1997. "On Stigma and Its Consequences: Evidence from a Longitudinal Study of Men with Dual Diagnoses of Mental Illness and Substance Abuse." *Journal of Health and Social Behavior* 38: 177–190.

Lipsitz, G. 1995. "The Possessive Investment in Whiteness: Racialized Social Democracy and the 'White' Problem in American Studies." *American Quarterly* 47, 369–387.

Lister, Ruth. 2004. *Poverty.* Cambridge: United Kingdom: Polity Press.

Liu, Xiaoru, and Howard Kaplan,. 2001. "Role Strain and Illicit Drug Use: The Moderating Influence of Commitment to Conventional Values." *Journal of Drug Issues* 31 (4), 833–856.

Lowie, Robert Harry. 1919. *The Tobacco Society of the Crow Indians.* New York: The Trustees.

———. 1983. *The Crow Indians.* Lincoln, NE: University of Nebraska Press.

Ludlow, Fitz Hugh. 1857. *The Hasheesh Eater: Being Passages from the Life of a Pythagorean.* New York: Harper and Brothers.

———. 1864. "John Heathburn's Title: A Tale in Two Parts." *Harper's New Monthly Magazine.* 28(165): 341–354 and 28(166):465–480.

———. 2009a. (original 1856). "The Apocalypse of Hasheesh." *Putman's Magazine* 8(48). Online at: http://www.erowid.org/culture/characters/ludlow_fitz_hugh/ludlow_fitz_hugh_article1.shtml. Accessed June 13, 2013.

———. 2009b. (original 1868). "Outlines of the Opium-Cure." In Horace Day, ed. *The Opium Habit.* New York: Harper and Brothers.

Luthar, S., and K. D'Avanzo. 1999. "Contextual Factors in Substance Use: A Study of Suburban and Inner-City Adolescents." *Developmental Psychopathology* 11:845–867.

Lynne-Landsman, Sarah D., Julia A. Graber, Tracy R. Nichols, and Gilbert Botvin,. 2011. "Is Sensation Seeking a Stable Trait or Does It Change over Time?" *Journal of Youth and Adolescence* 40 (1): 48–58.

Maher, Lisa. 1997. *Sexed Work: Gender, Race and Resistance in a Brooklyn Drug Market.* New York: Oxford University Press.

Makela, Klaus, Robin Room, E. Single, P. Sulkunen, and B. Walsh. 1981. *Alcohol, Society and State, Vol. 1: A Comparative Study of Alcohol Control.* Toronto: Addiction Research Foundation.

Malinowski, Bronislaw. 1922. *Argonauts of the Western Pacific: An Account of Native Enterprise and Adventure in the Archipelagos of Melanesian New Guinea.* London: Routledge and Kegan Paul.

Malloch, M. 2007. "Changing Focus: 'Drug-Related Crime' and the Criminological Imagination." In A. Barton, et al., eds, *Expanding the Criminological Imagination: Critical Readings in Criminology,* pp. 116–35. Cullompton: Willan Publishing.

Manhal-Baugus, Monique. 1998. "The Self-in-Relation Theory and Women for Sobriety:

Female-Specific Theory and Mutual Help Group for Chemically Dependent Women." *Journal of Addictions and Offender Counseling* 18 (2): 78–85.

Manning, P. 2007. "The Symbolic Framing of Drug Use in the News: Ecstasy and Volatile Substance Abuse in Newspapers." In P. Manning, ed. *Drugs and Popular Culture: Drugs, Media and Identity in Contemporary Society*, pp. 150–67. Cullompton: Willan Publishing.

Martin, M. 2007. "19th Century Illustrated Periodicals as International Means of Communication." *Revista Româna de Jurnalism si Comunicare* 2 (1): 52–57.

Mathiasen, Helle. 2009. "Dr. Jekyll Impaired." *American Journal of Medicine* 122(5): 492.

Mayfield, R. D., R. A., Harris, and M. A. Schuckit. 2008. "Genetic Factors Influencing Alcohol Dependence." *British Journal of Pharmacology* 154(2): 275–87.

McCoy, Alfred, Cathleen Read, and Leonard Adams. 1986. "The Mafia Connection." In Peter Park and Wasyl Matveychuk, eds. *Culture and Politics of Drugs*, pp.110–18. Dubuque, IA: Kendall/Hunt.

McCoy, Clyde, J. Bryan Page, Duane C. McBride, Brian Russe, and Richard Clayton. 1979. "Youth Opiate Use." In G. M. Beschner and A. S. Friedman, eds. *Youth Drug Abuse*, 353–376. Lexington, Massachusetts: Lexington Books.

Mcdermott, Peter. 1992. "Representations of Drug Users. Facts, Myths and Their Role in Harm Reduction Strategy." *Drug Text*. Online at: http://www.drugtext.org/Self-help-peer-support-and-outreach/representations-of-drug-users-facts-myths-and-their-role-in-harm-reduction-strategy.html.

McGovern, Patrick E. 2003. *Ancient Wine*. Princeton, NJ: Princeton University Press.

McGrath, E. 1981. "A Fraud in the Pulitzers." *Time* (Canadian edition) 117 (17): 74, 76, 78, 80.

McKenna, Terence. 1992. *Food of the Gods: A Radical History of Plants, Drugs, and Human Evolution*. New York: Rider & Co.

McLaughlin, D., and A. Long. 1996. "An Extended Literature Review of Health Professionals' Perceptions of Illicit Drugs and Their Clients Who Use Them. *Journal of Psychiatric and Mental Health Nursing* 3(5): 283–288.

Mencken, H. L. 1917. "The Divine Afflatus." *The New York Evening Mail*, November 16.

Miller, Jody, and Christopher Mullins. 2009. "Feminist Theories of Crime." In Francis T. Cullen, John Wright, and Kristie Blevins, eds., *Taking Stock: The Status of Criminological Theory*, 217–249. Piscateway, NJ: Transaction Publishers.

MIT Classics. 2011. Available at http://classics.mit.edu/Plato/symposium.html.

Mitchell, Stephen, translator. 2004. *Gilgamesh: A New English Version*. New York: Simon and Schuster.

MoJo News Team. 2012. "Full Transcript of the Mitt Romney Secret Video." *Mother Jones*. Available online at: http://www.motherjones.com/politics/2012/09/full-transcript-mitt-romney-secret-video#47percent.

Mokdad, Ali, James Marks, Donna Stroup, and Julie Gerberding. 2004. "Actual Causes of Death in the United States." 2000. *Journal of the American Medical Association* 291(10): 1238–1241.

Morgan, H. Wayne. 1981. *Drugs in America: A Social History 1800–1980*. Syracuse, NY: Syracuse University Press, 1981.

Morganthau, Tom, Mark Miller, Janet Huck, and Jeanne DeQuinne. 1986. "Kids and Cocaine: An Epidemic Strikes Middle America." *Newsweek*, March 17, 58–65.

Mortimer, W. Golden. 1974 [1901]. *History of Coca: "The Divine Plant" of the Incas*. San Francisco: Fitz Hugh Memorial Library Edition.

Mosher, Clayton, and Scott Atkins. 2007. *Drugs and Drug Policy: The Control of Consciousness Alteration.* Thousand Oaks, CA: Sage.

Mozes, Alan. 1999. "Poverty Has Greater Impact than Cocaine on Young Brains." *Reuters Health,* December 6.

Murphy, Dylan. 2013. "Money Laundering and the Drug Trade: The Role of the Banks." Global Research: Center for Research on Globalization. Available online at: http://www.globalresearch.ca/money-laundering-and-the-drug-trade-the-role-of-the-banks/5334205. Accessed June 14, 2013.

Murphy, Sheigla, and Paloma Sales. 2001. "Pregnant Drug Users: Scapegoats of the Reagan/Bush and Clinton Era Economics." *National Advocates for Pregnant Women.* Available online at: http://advocatesforpregnantwomen.org/main/publications/articles_and_reports/pregnant_drug_users_scapegoats_of_the_reaganbush_and_clinton_era_economics.php.

Murray, Nicolas. 2003. *Aldous Huxley.* New York: Abacus.

Musto, David F. 1987. *The American Disease: Origins of Narcotics Control.* New York: Oxford University Press.

Nadelmann, Ethan. 2007. "The Global War on Drugs Can Be Won." *Foreign Policy.* Online at: http://www.foreignpolicy.com/articles/2007/08/15/think_again_drugs.

Nahas, Gabriel G. 1973. *Marihuana—Deceptive Weed.* New York: Raven Press.

Najavits, Lisa, Roger Weiss, and Sarah Shaw. 1997. "The Link between Substance Abuse and Posttraumatic Stress Disorder in Women: A Research Review." *American Journal on Addictions* 6:273–283.

Nathan, Richard, and Thomas I. Gais. 1998. "The Early Findings about the Newest Federalism for Welfare." *Publius: The Journal of Federalism* 28(3): 95–103.

National Institute on Drug Abuse. 2012. "The Science of Drug Abuse and Addiction: What is Addiction." Available online at: http://www.drugabuse.gov/publications/media-guide/science-drug-abuse-addiction.

———. 2013. "Appropriations History Table." Available at http://www.drugabuse.gov/about-nida/legislative-activities/budget-information/fiscal-year-2012-budget-information/appropriations-history-table.

National Institutes of Health. 2013. "Appropriations 2000–2012." Available at http://officeofbudget.od.nih.gov/pdfs/FY12/Approp.%20History%20by%20IC)2012.pdf

Najavits, L. 2002 "'Seeking Safety': Therapy for Trauma and Substance Abuse." *Corrections Today* 64(6): 136–139.

Navarro, Vicente. 1986. *Crisis, Health, and Medicine: A Social Critique.* New York: Tavistock.

Needle, Richard, S. Coyle, H. Cesari, R. T. Trotter, M. Clatts, S. Koester, L. Price, et al. 1998. "HIV Risk Behaviors Associated with the Injection Process: Multiperson Use of Drug Injection Equipment and Paraphernalia in Injection Drug User Networks." *Substance Use and Misuse* 33(12): 2403–2423.

Needle, Richard, S. L. Coyle, S. G. Genser, and R. T. Trotter II, eds. 1995. *Social Networks, Drug Abuse, and HIV Transmission.* NIDA Research Monograph No. 151. NIH Pub. No. 95–3889. Washington, DC: Supt. of Docs., U.S. Govt. Printing Office.

Needle, Richard, Robert Trotter, Merrill Singer, Chris Bates, J. Bryan Page, David Metzger, and Louis Herns Marcelin. 2003. "Rapid Assessment of the HIV/AIDS Crisis in Racial and Ethnic Minority Communities: An Approach for Timely Community Interventions." *American Journal of Public Health* 93(6): 970–979.

Nelson-Zlupko, L., E. Kauffman, and M/ Dore.1995. "Gender Differences in Drug

Addiction and Treatment: Implications for Social Work Intervention with Substance-Abusing Women." *Social Work* 40(1): 45–54.

Nesse, R., and K. C. Berridge. 1997. "Psychoactive Drug Use in Evolutionary Perspective." *Science* 278 (5335): 63–66.

Netherly , P. J. 2010. "Early Holocene Coca Chewing in Northern Peru." *Antiquity* 84:939–953.

New York Times. 1976. " 'Welfare Queen' Becomes Issue in Reagan Campaign," 51.

Nin, Anaïs. 1977. *Delta of Venus Erotica.* Orlando, Florida: Harcourt, Inc.

———. 1994. *Children of the Albatross.* New York: Peter Owen.

Nisim, Sarit, and Benjamin Orly. 2010. "The Speech of Services Procurement: The Negotiated Order of Commodification and Dehumanization of Cleaning Employees." *Human Organization* 69(3):221–232.

Nunn, Kenneth. 2002. "Race, Crime and the Pool of Surplus Criminality: Or Why the 'War on Drugs' was a 'War on Blacks.'" *Journal of Gender, Race and Justice* 381:384–445.

Office of National Drug Control Policy. 2012. "Marijuana Legalization." Available online at: http://www.whitehouse.gov/ondcp/ondcp-fact-sheets/marijuana-legalization.

Orcutt, James, and J. Blake Turner. 1993. "Shocking Numbers and Graphic Accounts: Quantified Images of Drug Problems in the Print Media." *Social Problems* 40(2): 190–206.

Osio, Patrick. 2008. "U.S. Drug Users: Main Cause for Mexico's Bloodbath." New America Media. Online at: http://news.newamericamedia.org/news/view_article.html?article_id=759cac0f65d3b6b9db607bc793933172. Accessed August 8, 2013.

Ostrow, Ronald. 1990. "Casual drug users should be shot, Gates says." *Los Angeles Times,* September 6. Online at: http://articles.latimes.com/1990-09-06/news/mn-983_1_casual-drug-users. Accessed June 2, 2012.

Page, J. Bryan. 1983. "The Amotivational Syndrome Hypothesis and the Costa Rica Study: Relationships between Methods and Results." *Journal of Psychoactive Drugs* 15(4): 261–267.

———. 1989. Personal communication.

———. 1990. "Streetside Drug Use among Cuban Drug Users in Miami, Florida." In R. Glick and J. Moore, eds, *Drug Use in Hispanic Communities,* pp. 169–191. New Brunswick, NJ: Rutgers University Press.

———. 1993. "To Own the Streets: Implications of Approaches to Studying Drug Use in Dade County, Florida." Paper presented at the annual meetings of the American Anthropological Association, November 17–21, Washington, D.C.

———. 1997. "Needle Exchange and Reduction of Harm: An Anthropological view." *Medical Anthropology* 13:1–21.

———. 1999. "Historical Overview of Other Abusable Drugs." In R. T. Ammerman, P. J. Ott., and R. E. Tarter, eds, *Prevention and Societal Impact of Drug and Alcohol Abuse,* pp. 47–63. Mahwah, N. J.: L. Erlbaum Associates.

Page, J. Bryan, and William E. Carter. 1980. "Smoking Environment and Effects." In W.E. Carter, ed. *Cannabis in Costa Rica.* Philadelphia: ISHI Press, pp. 116–144.

Page, J. Bryan, and Jose Salazar Fraile. 1997. "Jones and Mono: Withdrawal and Urgency in HIV Risk." Paper presented at the annual meetings of the American Anthropological Association, Washington, D.C., November 17–21.

Page, J. Bryan, and Renee Llanusa-Cestero. 2006. "Changes in the Get-off: Social Process and Intervention in Risk Locales." *Substance Use and Misuse* 41(6–7), 1017–1028, 2006.

Page J. Bryan, and M. J. Miguez-Burbano. 1999. "Parenteral Alcohol Use in Colombia: Warning of a Future Trend?" *Medical Anthropology* 15(4): 1–13.

Page, J. Bryan and Merrill Singer. 2010. *Comprehending Drug Use: Ethnographic Research at the Social Margins.* Brunswick, NJ: Rutgers University Press.

Page, J. Bryan, Dale D. Chitwood, Prince C. Smith, Normie Kane, and Duane C. McBride. 1990. "Intravenous Drug Abuse and HIV Infection in Miami." *Medical Anthropology Quarterly* 4(1): 56–71.

Page, J. Bryan, Jack M. Fletcher, and William R. True. 1988. "Psychosociocultural Perspectives in Chronic Cannabis Use: The Costa Rican Follow-up." *Journal of Psychoactive Drugs* 20(1): 57–65.

Page, J. Bryan, P. Shapshak, E. M. Duran, G. Even, I. Moleon-Borodowski, and R. Llanusa-Cestero. 2006. "Detection of HIV-1 in Injection Paraphernalia: Risk in an Era of Heightened Awareness." *AIDS Patient Care* 20(8): 576–585.

Page, J. Bryan, Prince C. Smith, and Normie Kane. 1990a. "Shooting Galleries, Their Proprietors, and Implications for Prevention of AIDS." *Journal of Drug Issues* 5(1/2): 69–85.

Page, J. Bryan, Prince C. Smith, and Normie Kane. 1990b. "Venous Envy: The Importance of Having Usable Veins." *Journal of Drug Issues* 20(2):291–308.

Parker, Howard, Judith Aldridge, F. Measham. 1998. *Illegal Leisure: The Normalization of Adolescent Recreational Drug Use.* London: Routledge.

Parker, Howard, Lisa Williams, and Aldridge, Judith. 2002. "The Normalization of 'Sensible' Recreational Drug Use: Further Evidence from the North West England Longitudinal Study." *Sociology* 36(4): 941–964.

Parramore, Lynn Stuart. 2012. "Forbes 400 List Reveals Why the Greedy Rich Fully Deserve Your Contempt—And Jesus's." AlterNet. Available online at: http://www.alternet.org/economy/forbes-400-list-reveals-why-greedy-rich-fully-deserve-your-contempt-and-jesuss?page=0%2C0.

Paseos Amazónicos. 2013. "Shamanism Program." Available at http://www.paseosamazonicos.com/.

Pennock, Pamela. 2007. *Advertising Sin and Sickness.* DeKalb: Northern Illinois University Press.

Pepper, Art and Laurie Pepper. 1984. *Straight Life: The Story of Art Pepper.* New York: Da Capo Press.

Peretti-Watel. Patrick. 2003. "Heroin users as 'Folk Devils' and French Public Attitudes toward Public Health Policy." *International Journal of Drug Policy* 14(4): 321–329.

Petersen, Robert C., and Richard C. Stillman. 1978. *PCP Phencyclidine Abuse: An Appraisal.* Rockville, MD: NIDA Monograph # 21.

Phillips, Rod. 2000. *A Short History of Wine.* New York: Ecco, an Imprint of Harper Collins Publishers.

Piven, Frances Fox, and Richard Clowar. 2003. *Welfare Reform and Low Wage Labor Markets in The New Poverty Studies.* New York University Press.

Plant, Sadie. 1999. *Writings on Drugs.* London: Faber and Faber.

Poe, Edgar Allen. 1838. "Ligeia." *American Museum of Science, Literature and the Arts* 1(1): 25–37.

Pollack, Harold, Sheldon Danziger, Rukmalie Jayakody, and Kristen Seefeldt, 2001. "Substance Use among Welfare Recipients: Trends and Policy Responses." Available online at: http://www.fordschool.umich.edu/research/poverty/pdf/jcpr_pollack.pdf.

Pynchon, Thomas. 1966. *The Crying of Lot 49.* New York: J. B. Lippincott.

Rapping, Elaine. 1997. *The Culture of Recovery: Making Sense of the Self-Help Movement in Women's Lives.* Boston: Beacon Press.

Reese, Stephen, and Danielian, Lucig. 1988. "Intermedia Influence on the Drug Issue:

Converging on Cocaine." In Pamela Shoemaker, eds. *Communication Campaigns about Drugs: Government, Media, and the Public*. Hillsdale, NJ: Lawrence Erlbaum, 29–45.

Reinarman, Craig, and Harry Levine. 1989. "The Crack Attack: Politics and Media in America's Latest Drug Scare." In J. Best, ed. *Images and Issues: Typifying Contemporary Social Problems*. New York: Aldine De Gruyer.

Reinarman, Craig, and Harry Levine, 1997. "Crack in Context: America's Latest Demon Drug." In Craig Reinarman and Harry Levine, eds. *Crack In America: Demon Drugs and Social Justice*. Berkeley: University of California Press, 1–17.

Rettig, R., M. Torres, and G. Garrett. 1977. *Manny: A Criminal-Addict's Story*. Atlanta, GA: Houghton Mifflin, Review Press.

Riggins, Stephen, ed. 1997. *The Language and Politics of Exclusion: Others in Discourse*. Thousand Oaks, CA: Sage Publications.

Riggs, Mike. 2012. "4 Industries Getting Rich Off the Drug War." Available on line at: http://reason.com/archives/2012/04/22/4-industries-getting-rich-off-the-drug-w/2.

Riley, K. 1997. *Crack, Powder Cocaine, and Heroin: Drug Purchase and Use Patterns in Six US Cities*. Washington, DC: National Institute of Justice and Office of National Drug Control Policy.

Ripoll, Carme, José Salazar, and J. Bryan Page. 2002. "Drug-Using Sex Workers in the Streets of Valencia." *Journal of Ethnicity and Substance Abuse* 1(4): 1–27.

Rivera, M., A.. Aufderheide, L. W. Cartmell, C. M. Torres, and O. Langsjoen. 2005. "Antiquity of Coca-Leaf Chewing in the South Central Andes: A 3,000 Year Archaeological Record of Coca-Leaf Chewing from Northern Chile." *J. Psychoactive Drugs* 37 (4): 455–458.

Rodin, A. 1981. "Infants and Gin Mania in 18th-Century London." *Journal of the American Medical Association* 245(12): 1237–1239.

Rogak, Lisa. 2010. *Haunted Heart: The Life and Times of Stephen King*. New York: St. Martin's Griffin.

Rosen, Christine. 2005. "The Image Culture." *The New Atlantis: A Journal of Technology and Society*. Available at: http://www.thenewatlantis.com/publications/the-image-culture. Accessed April 30, 2011.

Rosenbaum, Marsha. 1981. *Women on Heroin*. New Brunswick, NJ: Rutgers University Press.

Rosenbaum, Milton, Phillip Piker, and Henry Lederer. 1940. "Delirium Tremens: A Study of Various Methods of Treatment." *American Journal of Medical Sciences* 200(5): 677–688.

Ross, Susan. 2011a. "Marking and Demarking: Images, Narratives, and Identities." In Susan Ross and Park Lestor, eds. *Images that Injure: Pictorial Stereotypes in the Media*, Santa Barbara: Praeger, 5–8.

Ross, Susan. 2011b. "Introduction." In Susan Ross and Park Lestor, eds. *Images that Injure: Pictorial Stereotypes in the Media*. Santa Barbara: Praeger, 1–4.

Rozen, David. 2007. "Anthropological and Public Health Perspectives on Social Inequality, Poverty, and Health." *Practicing Anthropology* 29(4): 39–42.

Rubin, Vera. 1975. "The 'Ganja Vision' in Jamaica." In Vera Rubin, ed. *Cannabis and Culture*. The Hague: Mouton, 257–265.

Rubin, Vera, and Lambros Comitas 1975. *Ganja in Jamaica*. The Hague, Netherlands: Mouton.

Rubin, Vera, and Comitas Lambros. 1983. "Cannabis, Society and Culture." In Maureen Kelleher, Bruce MacMurray, and Thomas Shapiro, eds. Dubuque, IA: Kendall/Hunt, 212–18.

Rush, Benjamin. 1786. *An Enquiry into the Effects of Spirituous Liquors upon the Human Body, and Their Influence upon the Happiness of Society.* [microform] [New York : Readex Microprint, 1985] 11 x 15 cm. (Early American imprints. First series ; no. 22865; 44963.

Sabelli, Michael. 2013. *Ryszard Kapuściński's Discourse on the Other: Literary Reportage's Perspective of Reality. Otherness: Essays and Studies* 3(2): 1–26.

Saïd, Edward. 1978. *Orientalism.* New York: Vintage Books.

Salinger, Sharon V. 2002. *Taverns and Drinking in Early America.* Baltimore, MD: Johns Hopkins University Press.

Sanders, Jolene 2009. *Women in Alcoholics Anonymous: Recovery and Empowerment.* Boulder, CO: First Forum Press.

Saxe, L., C. Kadushin, E. Tighe, D. Rindskopf, and A. Beveridge. 2001a. *National Evaluation of the Fighting Back Program: General Population Surveys, 1995–1999.* New York: City University of New York Graduate Center.

Saxe, L., C. Kadushin, A. Beveridge, D. Livert, E. Tighe, Elizabeth, D. Rindskopf, and J. Ford. 2001b. "The Visibility of Illicit Drugs: Implications for Community-Based Drug Control Strategies." *American Journal of Public Health* 91: 1987–1994.

Scarborough, John. 2010. *Pharmacy and Drug Lore in Antiquity.* Burlington, VT: Ashgate Publishing Company.

Schawlbe, Michael, Sandra Godwin, Daphne Holden, Douglas Schrock, Shealy Thompson, and Michele Wolkomir. 2000. "Generic Processes in the Reproduction of Inequality: An Interactionist Analysis." *Social Forces* 79(2): 419–453.

Schensul, Jean, Cristina Huebner, Merrill Singer, Lorie Broomhall, and Pablo Feliciano. 2000. "The High, the Money, and the Fame: The Social Context of 'New marijuana' Use among Urban Youth." *Medical Anthropology* 18:389–414.

Schultes, Richard Evans. 1938. "The Appeal of Peyote (Lophophora williamsii) as a Medicine." *American Anthropologist* 40(4): 698–715.

Schultes, Richard Evans. 1976. *Hallucinogenic Plants.* New York: Golden Press. Rotterdam, Netherlands: A. A. Balkema.

Schultes, Richard Evans. 1993. "Amazonian Ethnobotany and the Search for New Drugs." Ciba Foundation Symposium: Ethnobotany and the Search for New Drugs 185: 106–112.

Schur, Edwin. 1971. *Labeling Deviant Behavior: Its Sociological Implications.* New York: Harper & Row Publishers.

Scott, J. 1969. *The White Poppy.* New York: Harper and Row.

Seddon, Toby. 2010. *A History of Drugs.* New York: Routledge.

Sennett, Richard, and Jonathan Cobb. 1972. *The Hidden Injuries of Class.* New York: Vintage Books.

Sewell, R. Andrew, James Poling, and Mehmet Sofuoglu. 2009. "The Effect of Cannabis Compared with Alcohol on Driving." *American Journal on Addictions* 18(3): 185–193.

Shafer, R. P., D. Farnsworth, H. Brill, T. L. Carter, J. G. Cooney, C. O. Galvin, J. . Howard, H. E. Hughes, J. K. Javits, P. G. Rogers, M. H. Seevers, J. T. Ungerleider, and M. Ware. 1972. *Marihuana: A Signal of Misunderstanding. The Official Report of the National Commission on Marihuana and Drug Abuse.* New York: New American Library.

Siegel, Ronald. 2005. *Intoxication: The Universal Drive for Mind-Altering Substances.* Rochester, VT: Park Street Press.

Simmons, Janie, and Merrill Singer. 2006. "I Love You ... and Heroin: Care and Collusion among Drug-using Couples." *Substance Abuse Treatment, Prevention, and Policy* 1(7), online journal at: http://www.substanceabusepolicy.com/content/1/1/7.

Simon, David. 2008. "Interview by Bill Moyers." *Bill Moyer's Journal.* Available at http://www.pbs.org/moyers/journal/04172009/transcript1.html.

Singer, Merrill. 1986. "Toward a Political Economy of Alcoholism: The Missing Link in the Anthropology of Drinking Behavior." *Social Science and Medicine* 23(2): 113–130.

————. 1993. "Knowledge for Use: Anthropology and Community-Centered Substance Abuse Research." *Social Science and Medicine* 37(1): 15–26.

————. 1994. "AIDS and the Health Crisis of the U.S. Urban Poor: The Perspective of Critical Medical Anthropology." *Social Science and Medicine* 39(7): 931–948.

————. 1996a. "The evolution of AIDS work in a Puerto Rican community organization." *Human Organization* 55(1): 67–75.

————. 1996b. "A dose of drugs, a touch of violence, a case of AIDS: Conceptualizing the SAVA syndemic." *Free Inquiry in Creative Sociology* 24(2): 99–110.

————. 2004. "Why Is It Easier to Get Drugs than Drug Treatment?" In Arachu Castro and Merrill Singer, eds.*Unhealthy Health Policy: A Critical Anthropological Examination.* Walnut Creek, CA: Altamira Press, 287–303.

————. 2006. *The Face of Social Suffering: Life History of a Street Drug Addict.* Prospect Heights, IL: Waveland Press.

————. 2007. "Poverty, Welfare Reform and the 'Culture of Wealth.'" *Practicing Anthropology* 29(4): 43–45.

————. 2008. *Drugging the Poor: Legal and Illegal Drug Industries and the Structuring of Social Inequality.* Prospect Heights, IL: Waveland Press.

————. 2012. "Anthropology and Addiction: An Historic Review." *Addiction* 107(10): 1745–1755.

Singer, Merrill, and Mirhej, Greg. 2004. "The Understudied Supply Side: Public Policy Implications of the Illicit Drug Trade in Hartford, CT." *Harvard Health Policy Review* 5(2): 36–47.

Singer, Merrill, and Mirhej, Greg. 2006. *High Notes: The Role of Drugs in the Making of Jazz. Journal of Ethnicity and Substance Abuse* 5(4): 1–38.

Singer, Merrill, Pamela Erickson, Louise Badiane, R. Diaz, D. Ortiz, Traci Abraham, and Anna Marie Nicolaysen, 2006. "Syndemics, Sex and the City: Understanding Sexually Transmitted Disease in Social and Cultural Context." *Social Science and Medicine* 63(8): 2010–2021.

Singer, Merrill, Elsa Huertas, and Glenn Scott. 2000. "Am I My Brother's Keeper: A Case Study of the Responsibilities of Research." *Human Organization.* 59(4): 389–400.

Singer, Merrill, Greg Mirhej, Susan Shaw, Cristine Huebner, Julie Eiserman, Raul Pino, and J. Garcia. 2005. "When the Drug of Choice Is a Drug of Confusion: Embalming Fluid Use in Inner City Hartford, CT." *Journal of Ethnicity and Substance Abuse* 4(2): 71–96.

Singer, Merrill, Hassan Saleheen, Greg Mirhej, and Claudia Santelices. 2006. "Research Findings on Drinking among Street Drug Users." *American Anthropologist* 108(3): 502–506.

Singer, Merrill, Glen Scott, Scott Wilson, Delia Easton, and Margaret Weeks. 2001. "'War Stories': AIDS Prevention and the Street Narratives of Drug Users." *Qualitative Health Research* 11(5): 589–611.

Singer, Merrill, William Tootle and Joy Messerschmitt. 2013. "Living in an Illegal Economy: The Small Lives that Create Big Bucks in the Global Drug Trade." *School of Advanced International Studies Review of International Affairs (SAIS Review)* 33(1): 121–133.

Smith, Keven. 2004. "The Politics of Punishment: Evaluating Political Explanations of Incarceration Rates." *The Journal of Politics* 66(3): 925–938.

Smith, Phillip. 2012. "This Week's Corrupt Cops Stories. Stop the Drug War. Com." Online at: http://stopthedrugwar.org/taxonomy/term/27.

Standage, Tom. 2005. *A History of the World in 6 Glasses.* New York: Walker & Company.

Starks, Michael. 1982. *Cocaine Fields and Reefer Madness: An Illustrated History of Drugs in the Movies.* New York: Cornwall Books.

Stephens, R. 1991. *The Street Addict Role: A Theory of Heroin Addiction.* Albany, NY: State University of New York Press.

Stevenson, Robert Louis. 1886. *Strange Case of Dr. Jekyll and Mr. Hyde.* London: Longmanns, Green and Co.

Stratton, John. 1973. "Cops and Drunks: Police and Actions in Dealing with Indian Drunks." *The International Journal of the Addictions* 8(4): 613–621.

Substance Abuse and Mental Health Services Administration. 2008. "Results from the 2007 National Survey on Drug Use and Health: National Findings" (No. SMA 08-4343). Rockville, MD: Office of Applied Studies.

Sullivan, Roger, Edward Hagen, , and Peter Hammerstein, 2008. "Revealing the Paradox of Drug Reward in Human Evolution." *Proceedings of the Royal Society B-Biological Sciences* 275 (1640): 1231–1241.

Sutherland, John. 2001. *Last Drink to LA.* London: Short Books.

Swartz, J., A. Lurigio, and P. Goldstein. 2000. "Severe Mental Illness and Substance Use Disorders among Former Supplemental Security Income Beneficiaries for Drug Addiction and Alcoholism." *Archives of General Psychiatry* 57(7): 701–707.

Syal, Rajeev. 2009. "Drug Money Saved Banks in Global Crisis, Claims UN Advisor." *The Guardian.* Online at: http://www.guardian.co.uk/global/2009/dec/13/drug-money-banks-saved-un-cfief-claims. Accessed June 14, 2013.

Syvertsen, Jennifer Leigh. 2012. "Love and Risk? Intimate Relationships among Female Sex Workers Who Inject Drugs and Their Non-Commercial Partners in Tijuana, Mexico." A dissertation submitted in partial fulfillment of the requirements for the degree of Doctor of Philosophy, Department of Anthropology, College of Arts and Sciences, University of South Florida.

Szymanski, Ann-Marie. 2003. *Pathways to Prohibition: Radicals, Moderates, and Social Movement Outcomes.* Durham, NC: Duke University Press.

Taylor. Stuart. 2008. "Outsiders: Media Representations of Drug Use." *The Journal of Community and Criminal Justice* 55(4): 369–387.

Tepperman, Jean. 1998. "Welfare Reform Pioneers: What Can We Learn from States That Started Early with Aggressive Welfare-to-Work Policies?" In *Children's Advocate.* Berkeley, CA: Action Alliance for Children.

Thoman, Elizabeth. 1992. "Rise of the Image Culture: Re-Imagining the American Dream." CI 57 (Winter). Available online at: http://www.medialit.org/reading-room/rise-image-culture. Accessed April 30, 2011.

Thomas, Piri. 1967. *Down These Mean Streets.* New York: Vintage.

Thompson, Hunter. 1967. *Hell's Angels: The Strange and Terrible Saga of the Outlaw Motorcycle Gangs.* New York: Random House.

———. 1998 [1971] *Fear and Loathing in Las Vegas: A Savage Journey to the Heart of the American Dream.* New York: Vintage.

———. 2012. "BrainyQuote.com," Xplore Inc. Available online at: http://www.brainyquote.com/quotes/quotes/h/huntersth109598.html, accessed December 23, 2012.

Tonry, Michael. 1996. *Malign Neglect: Race, Crime, and Punishment in America.* Oxford: Oxford University Press.

Tortu, S., J. McMahon, E. Pouget, and R. Hamid. 2004. "Sharing of Noninjection Drug-Use Implements as a Risk Factor for Hepatitis C." *Substance Use and Misuse* 39(2): 211–224.

Townsend, Mark. 2008. "Drugs in Literature: A Brief History." *The Guardian*, November 15. Online at: http://www.guardian.co.uk/society/2008/nov/16/drugs-history-literature.

Trancas, B., N. Santos, and L. Patricio. 2008. "The Use of Opium in Roman Society and the Dependence of Princeps Marcus Aurelius." *Acta Medica Portuguesa* 21(6): 581–590.

Trojanowicz, Robert. 1991. *Community Policing and the Challenge of Diversity*. East Lansing, MI: The National Center for Community Policing, Michigan State University.

True, Willaim, J. Bryan Page, M. Hovey. and Paul Doughty. 1980. "Marijuana and User Lifestyles." In W.E. Carter, ed. *Cannabis in Costa Rica*. Philadelphia: ISHI Press, 98–115.

Tsuang M., M. Lyons, J. Meyer, T. Doyle, S. Eisen, J. Goldberg, W. True, N. Lin, R. Toomey, and L. Eaves. 1998. "Co-occurrence of Abuse of Different Drugs in Men." *Archives of General Psychiatry* 55:967–972.

Tyrrell, Ian. 1991. *Woman's World/Woman's Empire: The Woman's Christian Temperance Union in International Perspective, 1880–1930*. Chapel Hill: University of North Carolina Press.

Tyrrell, Ian. 2010. *Reforming the World*. Princeton, New Jersey: Princeton University Press.

U.S. Congress. 1977, *House Select Committee on Narcotics Abuse and Conrol. Southeast Asian Narcotics. Hearings, 95th Congress, Ist session*. Washington, D.C.: U.S. Government Printing Office.

Ulleland, Christy 1972. "Offspring of Alcoholic Mothers." *Annals of The New York Academy of Sciences* 197:167–168.

USA Today. 2012. "Editorial: Drug Testing Welfare Applicants Nets Little." Available online: http://usatoday30.usatoday.com/news/opinion/editorials/story/2012-03-18/drug-testing-welfare-applicants/53620604/1.

Vaillant, George E. 1983. *The Natural History of Alcoholism*. Cambridge, MA: Harvard University Press.

Verdejo-Garcia, Antonio, Lawrence, Andrew and Clark, Luke. 2008. "Impulsivity as a vulnerability marker for substance-use disorders: review of findings from high-risk research, problem gamblers and genetic association studies." *Neuroscience and Biobehavioral Reviews* 32(4): 777-810.

Van Radowitz, John. 2010. "Drunk Writers Were Better Sober Says Psychiatrist." *The Independent*. June 25. On line at: http://www.independent.co.uk/news/science/drunk-writers-were-better-sober-says-psychiatrist-2010053.html.

Vargas, Theresa. 2010. "Once Written Off, 'Crack Babies,' have Grown into Success Stories." April 18. *The Washington Post*. Available online at: http://www.washingtonpost.com/wp-dyn/content/article/2010/04/15/AR2010041502434.html

Virginia Department of Mental Health, Mental Retardation and Substance Abuse Services. 2004. "Gender Differences and Their Implications for Substance Abuse Disorder Treatment. Reviews to Use." Available online at: www.dbhds.virginia.gov/documents/OSAS-REGenderSpecificSATX.doc. Accessed June 11, 2013.

Vulliamy, Ed. 2008. "Global Banks are the Financial Services Wing of the Drug Cartels." *The Guardian*, July 21. Available online at http://www.guardian.co.uk/world/2012/jul/21/drug-cartels-banks-hsbc-money-laundering.

Wacquant, Loïc. 2001. "Deadly Symbiosis: When Ghetto and Prison Meet and Mesh." *Punishment & Society* 3(1): 95–133.

Walitzer, Kimberly and Sher, Kenneth. 1996. "A Prospective Study of Self-Esteem and Alcohol Use Disorders in Early Adulthood: Evidence for Gender Differences." *Alcoholism: Clinical and Experimental Research* 20(6): 1118-1124.

Wal-Mart Watch. 2012. "Wal-Mart Employees Speak Out." Available online at: http://walmartspeakout.com/.

Wallace, J., T. Brown, J. Bachman, and T. Laveist, 2003. "The Influence of Race and Religion on Abstinence from Alcohol, Cigarettes and Marijuana among Adolescents." *Journal of Studies on Alcohol* 64:843–848.

Waterston, Alysse. 1993. *Street Addicts in the Political Economy.* Philadelphia: Temple University Press.

Weaver, Vesla, and Amy Lerman. 2010. *Political Consequences of the Carceral State. American Political Science Review* 104(14): 817–833.

Weis, Lois. 1995. "Identity Formation and the Processes of 'Othering': Unraveling Sexual Threads." *Educational Foundations* 9(1): 17–33.

West, Cornel. 1993. *Prophetic Thought in Post Modern Times: Beyond EuroCentricism.* Monroe, ME: Common Courage Press.

Weston, Bruce. 2010. "Decriminalizing Poverty." *The Nation.* On line at: http://www.thenation.com/article/157007/decriminalizing-poverty.

Whitehead, Tom. 2009. "Drug Rehabilitation for Offenders a Waste of Time, Says Judge." *London Telegraph,* January 7. Available at http://www.telegraph.co.uk/news/uknews/law-and-order/4162834/Drug-rehabilitation-for-offenders-a-waste-of-time-says-judge.html.

Wight, William. 1845?. *Common Sense: A Word to Those Who Do Not Think by Proxy.* Glasgow: Office of the Scottish Temperance League. http://find.galegroup.com/mome/infomark.do?&contentSet=MOMEArticles&type=multipage&tabID=T001&prodId=MOME&docId=U3606532590&source=gale&userGroupName=miami_richter&version=1.0&docLevel=FASCIMILE.

Wilbert, Johannes. 1972. "Tobacco and Shamanistic Ecstasy among the Warao Indians of Venezuela." In P. T. Furst, ed. *Flesh of the Gods: The Ritual Use of Hallucinogens.* Prospect Heights, IL: Waveland Press, 136–184.

Wilde, Oscar. 1890. "The Picture of Dorian Gray." *Lippincott's Monthly Magazine,* July: 1–100.

Williams, T. 1992. *Crackhouse: Notes From the End of the Line.* New York, NY: Penguin Books.

Wills, David. 2011. "The Weird Cult: William S. Burroughs and Scientology." *Beatdom Literary Journal.* Available on line at: http://www.beatdom.com/?p=1373.

Windsor, Lilliane, and Eloise Dunap. 2010. "What Is Substance Use About? Assumptions in New York's Drug Policies and the Perceptions of African Americans Who are Low-Income and Using Drugs." *Journal of Ethnicity in Substance Abuse,* 9:64–87.

Wolf, Eric. 1982. *Europe and the People Without History.* Berkeley: University of California Press.

Woods, Crawford. 1972. "The Best Book on the Dope Decade." *The New York Times Review of Books,* July 23. Available online at: http://www.nytimes.com/books/98/11/29/specials/thompson-vegas.html.

World Health Organization. 2004. *Global Status Report on Alcohol.* Geneva: World Health Organization Department of Mental Health and Substance Abuse.

Wright, Daniel. 1994. "The Prisonhouse of My Disposition: A Study of the Psychology of Addiction in Dr. Jekyll and Mr. Hyde." *Studies in the Novel.* 26.(3): 254–267.

Wright, Paul. 2013. "The Crime of Being Poor." *Prison Legal News.* Online at: https://www.

prisonlegalnews.org/(X(1)S(muq1sonbeyu1on45rh0uea45))/displayArticle.aspx?
articleid=6070&AspxAutoDetectCookieSupport=1. Accessed June 11, 2013.

Wu, Li-Tzy, Woody, George, Yang, Chongming, Pan, Jeng-Jong, and Blzaer, Dan. 2011. "Racial/Ethnic Variations in Substance-Related Disorders Among Adolescents in the United States." *Archives of General Psychiatry* 68(11):1176–1185.

X, Malcolm. 1987 [1977]. *The Autobiography of Malcolm X.* New York: Random House Publishing Group.

Yongming, Zhou. 1999. *Anti-drug Crusades in Twentieth-Century China: Nationalism, History and State Building.* Lanham, MA: Roman and Littlefield Publishers.

Young, J. 1973. "The Myth of the Drugtaker in the Mass Media." In S. Cohen and J. Young, eds. *The Manufacture of News.* London: Constable.

Zimmer, Lynn. 1992. "The Anti-Drug Semantic." Paper presented at the Drug Policy Foundation Conference, Washington, D.C.

Zinberg, N., and Andrew Weil. 1969. "Cannabis—1st Controlled Experiment." *New Society* 13(329): 84-86.

Zucchino, David. 1999. *Myth of the Welfare Queen: A Pulitzer Prize-Winning Journalist's Portrait of Women on the Line.* New York: Touchstone.

INDEX

ABOUT THE AUTHORS

J. Bryan Page, PhD, is professor and chair in the Department of Anthropology at the University of Miami. Research on people who engage in socially disapproved behaviors has dominated Bryan Page's professional activity for the last three decades. He has studied patterns of marihuana smoking, poly-drug consumption, self-injection, crack use, and sex trade. These studies have relied on a number of methods, including direct observation of risky behaviors, in-depth interviewing of drug users, qualitative analysis of textual materials, focus groups, survey methods, secondary data analysis, results of physical examinations, and laboratory techniques for determining immune status, viral load, and/or recent drug consumption. Dr. Page recently co-authored a book with Merrill Singer on the ethnographic study of drug use (August, 2010). He has conducted studies funded by the National Institute on Drug Abuse and the National Institute of Mental Health. His research experience in local neighborhoods uniquely equips him to help research teams to accomplish goals related to intervening at the community level and monitoring the impact of the intervention. Dr. Page's publications often address questions of community setting and approaches to finding specific populations in those settings. His recent work has emphasized the value of on-the-scene perspectives in the study of human behaviors such as formation of couples, seeking of health care, and uptake of tobacco use.

Merrill Singer, PhD, a medical and cultural anthropologist, is a Professor in the departments of Anthropology and Community Medicine, and a Senior Research Scientist at the Center for Health, Intervention and Prevention at the University of Connecticut. Additionally, he is affiliated with the Center for Interdisciplinary Research on AIDS at Yale University. Over his career, his research and writing have addressed HIV/AIDS in highly vulnerable and disadvantaged populations, illicit drug use and drinking behavior in light of political economy, community and structural violence, health disparities, and the political ecology of health. His research focuses especially on the nature and impact of both syndemics (interacting epidemics) and pluralea (intersecting ecocrises) on health. Dr. Singer has published over 260 articles and book chapters and has authored or edited 25 books. He is a recipient of the Rudolph Virchow Prize, the George Foster Memorial Award for Practicing

Anthropology, the AIDS and Anthropology Paper Prize, the Prize for Distinguished Achievement in the Critical Study of North America, and the Solon T. Kimball Award for Public and Applied Anthropology from the American Anthropological Association.